AFTER
BREAST
CANCER

AFTER BREAST CANCER

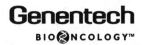

After Breast Cancer: Answers to The Questions You're Afraid to Ask
by Musa Mayer

Copyright © 2003 Musa Mayer. All rights reserved.
Printed in the United States of America

Published by O'Reilly Media, Inc., 1005 Gravenstein Hwy North,
Sebastopol, CA 95472.

Editor: Linda Lamb

Production Editor: Tom Dorsaneo

Cover Designer: Kristen Throop

Printing History: March 2003. First Edition.

Many of the designations used by manufacturers and sellers to distinguish their products
are claimed as trademarks. Where those designations appear in this book, and O'Reilly
Media, Inc. was aware of a trademark claim, the designations have been printed in
caps or initial caps.

This book is meant to educate and should not be used as an alternative for professional medical care. Although we have exerted every effort to ensure that the information presented is accurate at the time of publication, there is no guarantee that this
information will remain current over time. Appropriate medical professionals should
be consulted before adopting any procedures or treatments discussed in this book.

Library of Congress Cataloging-in-Publication Data:

Mayer, Musa
     After breast cancer: answers to the questions you're afraid to ask /
    Musa Mayer.
       p. cm – (Patient-centered guides)
    Includes index.
     1. Breast—Cancer—Relapse—Popular works. I. Title. II. Series.

RC280 B8M349 2003
616.99'449–dc21   2002193112

This book is printed on acid-free paper with 85% recycled content, 15%
post-consumer waste. O'Reilly Media, Inc. is committed to using paper
with the highest recycled content available consistent with high quality.

[M]

Who are they,
the two million strong?
They are you and me,
hand in hand.

Table of Contents

Introduction

THIS IS A DIFFERENT KIND OF BOOK for women diagnosed with breast cancer.

This book is about what happens *after* surgery, radiation and chemotherapy are over, and the uncertainty sets in. Maybe you are still in that vulnerable post-treatment period when everyone expects you to get back to life as usual. Or, maybe you are one or two or a few more years down the line, free of recurrence, but still worried about it, especially when you go back to see your oncologist or have tests done.

You may have some questions about the importance of follow-up testing to detect recurrence early. You may be wondering if your risk for recurrence changes over time, or what specific symptoms you should be looking for. You're probably not entirely sure how vigilant you should be. You almost certainly have concerns about what you would be facing, should you actually develop metastatic breast cancer. At a time when your doctors and family are advising you to think positively and turn your attention elsewhere, you may be secretly feeling anxious, upset, and alone with your fears.

This is a book that addresses these worries about recurrence directly, through information and the support of many women who have been there, just like you.

This book takes the position that for women diagnosed with breast cancer, coming to terms in a direct way with the fear of recurrence can become a crucial part of the recovery process.

A personal note

After Breast Cancer is my third book about breast cancer.

When I was diagnosed with Stage II breast cancer in 1989, I managed my fear and got back in control primarily through a search for information—not a simple task prior to the easy accessibility of the Internet. The patient pamphlets I found didn't give me the depth of information that I wanted, so I bought a medical text entitled, *Cancer of the Breast.* I recall sitting up night after night, absorbing what I could, a medical diction-ary by my side. By the day of my surgery, I had at least the beginnings of a grasp of the disease and what I would be facing. During that difficult time, a few women who had already com-pleted their treatment reached out to me with their stories about mastectomy, chemotherapy and reconstruction, and that helped, too, more than I can say.

Although I was already a writer, with a memoir published just the year before my diagnosis, two years passed before I was able to put my own cancer experience into words. After *Examining Myself: One Woman's Story of Breast Cancer Treatment and Recovery* was published in 1993, I joined the newly formed Breast-Cancer Mailing List on the Internet, a large international group of women and men who discuss all aspects of breast cancer via the daily exchange of e-mail (for more information, see *http://www .bclist.org*). I wanted to give back what had been given to me, to reach out to other newly diagnosed women with information and support.

My involvement with the Breast-Cancer Mailing List exposed me to the extraordinary wisdom, eloquence and candor of patients and their families who were having to cope with metastatic breast cancer and very high-risk primary breast cancer. These were stories that must be told, I decided, and so the idea for what became *Advanced Breast Cancer: A Guide to Living with Metastatic Disease* was born. Unlike my memoir, the book did not derive from personal experience, but rather focused on the realities of Stage III and IV breast cancer, offering stories, information and resources for a group of patients whose needs and perspectives have been sorely neglected.

My long-time fascination with medicine and scientific research, a career direction I'd never pursued, was reawakened by my own diagnosis and subsequent involvement with helping other women. Over the years since the publication of this second breast cancer book, I've become increasingly involved with patient advocacy and drug development, attending oncology conferences and closely following the research that holds the best promise of improvements in survival, especially for metastatic patients. Learning some of the basics of cell biology, epidemiology and clinical trials (with the help of the National Breast Cancer Coalition's excellent science training program for advocates, Project LEAD), has led to my work, more recently, as a Patient Representative/Consultant for the FDA, where I offer input from a patient perspective on drug development issues.

With this third book, I've tried to weave in the two threads that have been most important to me: both the medicine and science of breast cancer, and my own and others' stories that possess the power to heal, explain and counsel. The medical information offers information about recurrence. The personal stories, told in patients' own words, eloquently illustrate the complexity of the ways in which cancer can bring about change and lead us to new places in our lives.

This is my second book for the Patient-Centered Guides series, a growing resource library that embraces the powerful combination of personal stories and up-to-date medical information made comprehensible for patients.

Some passages from this book have been adapted from essays I've written over the past five years as a contributing Editor of *MAMM Magazine,* and for the *www.SusanLoveMD.com* website, here gratefully republished with permission.

Acknowledgements

For their invaluable help in critiquing this manuscript and ensuring its accuracy, I want to extend my heartfelt thanks to medical oncologists, Dr. George Sledge, Ballve-Lantero Professor of Oncology at the Indiana University School of Medicine; Dr. Clifford Hudis, Chief of the Breast Cancer Medical Service at Memorial Sloan-Kettering Cancer Center, and Dr. Bill Buchholz, author of *Live Longer, Live Larger*; to oncology nurse Kathleen Allen; to nuclear medicine techologist Toya Powell; and to fellow advocates Helen Schiff and Sara McKenna.

Without the encouragement and support of Linda Lamb, of Patient-Centered Guides at O'Reilly & Associates, this book would not have become a reality. I am grateful to Deanna Blevins, who guided the book through the hard work of editorial revision and production. By taking on the task of supervising a messy apartment renovation himself, my husband Tom made it possible for me to find the time and quiet to work on this book. Without his devoted support, I could never accomplish my advocacy work.

Most of all, I am grateful for the enthusiastic, thoughtful and generous cooperation of the 42 women and two men whose words serve to animate the pages of this book. This book is dedicated to their spirit and resilience.

CHAPTER 1

Two Million Strong

OVER TWO MILLION WOMEN diagnosed with invasive breast cancer at some time in their lives are alive today in the United States. This year alone, over 200,000 more newly diagnosed women will join them.

Although breast cancer "awareness" is now very much in the news, typically the media only focus on part of the story, usually on early detection and getting through the rigors of treatment. After that, we are expected to get on with our lives. We may expect this of ourselves.

But after treatment is over, women still think about breast cancer and its impact on their lives. We find that we've been changed by our experience—physically, emotionally and spiritually. We can't forget about it immediately, and we're not sure we really want to, anyway.

This chapter examines what women who have finished treatment are facing: what we've lost, what we fear about the future, and how we've changed. Just because the media and the public are not talking about the possibility of recurrence doesn't mean that it never enters our mind, even though we are symptom free and feel well.

Breast cancer, then and now

In 1989, when I was diagnosed, breast cancer was not often in the news. No longer the secret it had once been, in the 1970's and earlier, the disease was still kept quiet—apart from the occasional celebrity revelation. Advertising campaigns were not yet emblazoned with pink ribbons, and October felt like just another month.

Today, all this has changed dramatically. Breast cancer has become a perennial topic in the minds of American women. Hardly a week goes by without major news coverage relating to breast cancer, whether it's a new research finding or a controversy over screening. Periodicals, including women's magazines, now often run feature articles on breast cancer.

A quick search of the *New York Times* website reveals 319 references to breast cancer, including quite a few major articles, in just the past 30 days. Today, I counted 91 books that incorporated personal breast cancer stories in print from among the first 300 of nearly a thousand books in print on breast cancer.

Television and the print media feed us a steady stream of mostly hopeful news. We are besieged by charitable appeals, by walks and runs, by branded products and messages of early detection, breast self-examination and mammography. Women diagnosed with breast cancer have become a market force.

In part, this is because there are so many of us. Breast cancer is the most common cancer in women, afflicting nearly a third of all women living with cancer today in the United States. Incidence of invasive breast cancer has increased, according to 2002 estimates, to 203,500 women per year. An additional 54,300 cases of DCIS, *in situ* or non-invasive breast cancer are predicted this year.

Whatever advances have been made in treatment and early detection, breast cancer is still the second most common cause of cancer death in women. 39,600 American women will die of the disease this year, or 15 percent of the total 267,300 cancer deaths estimated in 2002 in the United States.

But the good news is that women who have had breast cancer are surviving in ever-increasing numbers, now estimated by the National Cancer Institute at well over two million alive today.[1]

If you are reading these words and have had breast cancer, you are part of the community that shares this bond.

You are one of the two million strong.

What's bothering us

If breast cancer "awareness" has been a public health goal, we've certainly succeeded. Pollsters tell us that breast cancer is now the most feared disease for American women, although heart disease takes many more lives. They tell us that women consistently overestimate their risk for breast cancer. "The positive effort to increase public awareness of breast cancer," lamented one public health official, "has had the unfortunate effect of distorting women's perceptions of breast cancer risk."[2]

The sheer numbers in the statistics above may seem remote and abstract, set beside the power of our personal stories—the kinds of stories we hear from family, friends, at work, and wherever we are in contact with other women. Everyone knows someone who has had breast cancer, and we've never been more open to talking about it.

But the new openness about breast cancer has been almost exclusively focused on the early detection, diagnosis and treatment of primary breast cancer. Decades ago, when breast cancer was still a shameful secret and American women were much more often diagnosed at later stages of the disease, this focus made real sense. When mammography became widely available, a massive public education effort was launched to help women detect their cancers early, at more curable stages.

But what of the two million women alive in America today who have already moved past early detection and treatment to the reality of living with a breast cancer diagnosis? For us, casual references to the future are often laden with meaning. We can't help wondering which verb tense to use to describe our current relationship with the disease.

A breast cancer patient named Martha expressed this struggle well.

> I remember once, while in the oncologist's waiting room, being asked by another patient what kind of cancer I had. I replied, "I have breast cancer." I was immediately corrected by my brother who said, "No, you had breast cancer." I didn't know how to feel about that. I do know he was trying to be reassuring and attempting to get me to see myself in a different light. Was the cancer really gone once I had the surgery? Did I have breast cancer or had I had breast cancer?

For years after my own diagnosis with breast cancer, I struggled with those verb tenses, too. I could claim neither answer as factually accurate. The reality was, I just didn't know. In the end, I settled for just telling people of my diagnosis. "But you're fine now?" they'd ask. "So far," I would answer.

The fact is, our issues change, once we're done with our treatment. In the midst of the annual pink ribbon campaigns for awareness and early detection, where are the resources for breast cancer survivors, whether they are six months, six years or sixteen years past diagnosis? And what is it we still need, anyway—from ourselves, from our doctors, and from one another?

Clearly, there is something about having had breast cancer that stays with many of us, preventing us from putting this illness out of our minds and into the past. From my own experience and that of the hundreds of women I've heard discussing these issues over the years, I believe that what's bothering us is fundamentally three-fold: what we've lost, what we fear and how we've changed.

What we've lost

Over time, our sense of what we have lost is very likely to become tempered—and even outweighed—by evidence of personal growth, as hard-won struggles lead to a new awareness of resilience and strength, a new sense of freedom, and new perspectives, as priorities are clarified and trivial involvements fall away.

No cancer survivor has to look very far to find inspirational accounts from other survivors reflecting on the gifts life-threatening illness has brought into their own lives. For this transformative power, we can be grateful. Where would we be without the innate capacity most of us possess to adapt to whatever life hands us, to turn adverse events into challenges, given the time to process what has happened to us, with the support of caring others?

The losses we feel are real, nonetheless, and must be acknowledged and given the honor of our compassionate attention, if we are to work through our feelings of grief and anger to achieve some sense of acceptance and move toward emotional recovery. This is the important work of breast cancer support groups all around the country. Ignoring this natural grieving process in an effort to move on prematurely, through suppressing emotion and forcing an optimism one does not yet feel, is likely to have emotional costs later on.

No one could provide a complete inventory of all the losses, short and longer term, that can accompany a diagnosis with breast cancer. For each of us, the fabric of loss will be different and changing.

Yet there are some common threads. We suffer physically as a result of surgery, chemotherapy and, if we are young enough, from chemopause, the sudden menopause brought on by chemotherapy. The effects of radiation treatment, and ongoing hormonal treatment take their toll. Even if we don't experience chemopause, or the many other short and longer-term side effects of treatment, or the sense of having been mutilated by surgery, we are still often left with a feeling that our bodies have betrayed us.

We may feel aged by the treatment in other ways, and suffer blows to our self-esteem and sense of attractiveness, libido, sexuality and sexual appeal. If we are young, we may face the loss of fertility. We often experience significant weight gain with chemotherapy. Even with the support of a loving and patient partner, these losses may be hard to bear, especially in the first few years after diagnosis. For women who are single, this can be especially devastating.

Long after my mastectomy had healed and the indignities of chemotherapy were over, I still found myself hot-flashing a dozen times a day, gaining weight, fighting depression and anxiety, hobbling around on aching knees. I remember one day confessing to my husband, in tears, that I felt like "damaged goods."

Anywhere that women gather to discuss breast cancer, you will hear variations on this theme of loss. Who else can we share our complaints with, if not one another? Who else could possibly understand? Our families feel helpless, and soon tire of hearing about our symptoms. Our doctors often minimize the toxicities of treatment, and have few solutions to offer. Placing the emphasis on its life-saving potential, they tend to downplay the physical changes the cancer therapy brings. We're grateful the treatment exists, of course, but that doesn't mean we haven't had to pay a stiff price.

What we fear

For many women with breast cancer, this is the first close brush with mortality. The reality of one's own death is suddenly very much closer, having moved from an abstract inevitability to a very real, possible outcome. Suddenly, with the words "You have cancer," one's sense of safety, security and optimism about life and the future is shaken. The world is revealed as unfair and unsafe, for many. This can turn out to be the most profound loss, the loss underlying all the other losses—the loss of innocence.

Uncertainty seems to dwell at the core of these feelings, and it's a process that can persist for years. The fragile tissue of hope can be rebuilt when there are no further problems, but may be shredded all over again when something else happens.

Three years after her initial diagnosis and treatment, Ruthe wrote of her own loss of innocence as she waited to find out if the new lump she'd found in her lumpectomy scar was a local recurrence of her breast cancer. Terrified once again, she was struggling to reach a state of acceptance.

> *I am no longer innocent. I now understand that it's possible for anyone, any healthy woman with no risk factors, to turn up with breast cancer. And I know that the chances this lump is malignant are much greater than they were with the first lump, because cancer has been in my body, presumably removed through lumpectomy, chemotherapy and radiation, but perhaps not completely. But I can still be a survivor, because to me the term means accepting reality without judgment.*

> *If I have cancer again, I simply do—it's a fact and there is no point railing about the unfairness of the universe. Whether or not I choose to see it as tragedy is my choice. As I said to my girlfriend, "If it turns out to be cancer, I can get those fake breasts I've always wanted."*

Even when there is no recurrence, the fear persists, affecting us in odd ways long after treatment is over, as this post from Nancy D illustrates.

> *In spite of my newfound (cautious) optimism I have this irrational thing about keeping around my wig and prosthesis. I really should donate them, but every time I think about it I start to get anxious. There is that little superstitious corner of my brain that says "Don't jinx it!" So I still have my wig—that I never wore because I only lost half of my hair—and I still have my prosthesis that I haven't needed since my TRAM reconstruction five years ago. Not only that, but I couldn't even use it if I had to have another mastectomy because it only fits the right side! So I keep them both on a shelf in my bedroom— and so far they've kept "it" away.*

In the early years after my diagnosis, I struggled with these issues as well. My life had never actually been fair or predictable. No one's ever is, though it certainly may seem so for long, blissful stretches, especially when one is young. The future could never be counted upon, not really. But I'd been living my life as if these illusions were true, and it wasn't easy to let go of them.

So I was no more prepared than anyone else is for living with the long-lasting fear of breast cancer recurrence, or the worry that would awaken me in the early hours before a doctor's appointment, or the misery of waiting for test results, or the sense of dread I felt when a woman I knew was diagnosed with metastatic disease, or when the words "died of breast cancer" leapt off the obituary page. Why was that rib beneath where my breast had been so tender to the touch? Could an afternoon's gardening possibly have caused the lower back pain that radiated down my leg, and why was the pain lasting for ten days? The cluster of red bumps near my scar had been there for an awfully long time, hadn't it? Should I call my oncologist? Should I ask to be tested? Was I just being alarmist?

This is the kind of internal dialogue that breast cancer patients live with in the months and years immediately following the end of treatment. These are the thoughts they learn not to share with their husbands and partners and children, for fear of worrying them or trying their patience. After some months of this nearly constant anxiety, like many women, I began to worry about my own emotional stability. I had always thought of myself as strong, adaptable, even somewhat stoic—the kind of person upon whom others relied when they were troubled. Yet here I was, crying at the drop of a hat, having trouble sleeping, obsessively thinking dark thoughts in the middle of the night. I wasn't getting on with my life at all. What was wrong with me?

How we've changed

So much changes with a cancer diagnosis, as Gaelyne conveyed in this message to the Breast-Cancer Mailing List.

> *When we are diagnosed, we are suddenly faced with our own mortality, which we might not have given much thought to until then. For awhile, we are cocooned in a surreal world with doctors appointments, chemo infusions, building right up to daily trips for radiation. Then suddenly the doctors smile kindly and tell you to go live the rest of your life. At the same time,*

friends and family are very caring and check in with
you to provide much needed support. When treatment
ends, our friends assume we're cured and then say silly
things like they can't believe how good we look.

Meanwhile our world and our outlook has
dramatically changed and it's as if the scaffolding were
pulled out from under us again. We feel vulnerable and
fear and anger creeps in.

I've healed physically from my mastectomy,
radiation and chemo, but there's still an awful lot of
emotional healing that's now happening. I find it very
reassuring to know that I'm not the only person
walking down this road.

After my own diagnosis, I longed to hear and read about what it had been like for other women who had been there before me. The power of stories and shared experience was clear to me even then, but in 1989 there just weren't many published stories to turn to. I am forever grateful to the small network of women who took me under their wings and told me what having breast cancer had been like for them. Their stories made me believe that I could do it, too, that I could find within myself the strength to get through the treatments I dreaded so much at first.

It wasn't until I joined a support group that I learned how common, even normal, my emotional reactions were. It took many months of sorting out my own feelings and hearing the experiences of others, to begin to grasp how much had changed in my life and in my psyche.

Since then, I've been privileged to witness this healing process at work again and again, as women reach out to one another through sharing their stories. The powerful medicine of sisterhood continues to work its quiet magic.

Public silence, private dread

Based on my own experiences, and what I've observed in hundreds of women and a few men with breast cancer whom I've had the pleasure of knowing over the years, I have come to believe that for many of us (but not all), our post-treatment needs are simple and straightforward: open discussion of our issues, access to good information, and contact with and support from others who have been there.

We need some process through which we can talk freely about what's worrying us, whatever it may be. This process can and should take a variety of forms, from the give and take that happens when a patient consults her doctor, to a conversation with a nurse who takes the time to listen, to patients sharing their experiences with one another in a waiting room, to calls and questions from friends and family members who care, and to writing in a journal, or painting, or making music. We need some way—preferably many ways—to come to terms with the complex and changing emotions and thoughts we are experiencing.

Open discussion is crucial for the simple reason that it almost always helps to express what bothers us, providing us with a way of working through what's on our minds. Openness to this on the part of others is not as easy to find as one might think. Among psychologically sophisticated people who have not themselves experienced cancer, the "fear factor" often seems to take over, leading to the usual recommendations to think positively and hope for the best that every cancer patient gets sick of hearing. Unfortunately, not talking about worries over recurrence doesn't make those feelings go away—would that it were that simple! Many women find themselves feeling alone with their fears. When the message from those around them, including their doctors, is to "put it behind you" and "not to worry," women will come to feel that any further discussion of recurrence, or fear of recurrence, is unwelcome.

We also need access to the best sources of information about the disease and its treatments that are out there—and they are out there. When I was diagnosed, it was hard to know where to look. There was no Internet, no *Dr. Susan Love's Breast Book*. Looking up medical research meant getting permission to visit a medical library.

Now almost everything we need to know is easily accessed from our own homes, online. Those without computers can visit their public libraries for access and help with finding what they need. Today, our problem is reversed. Rather than a scarcity of information, we suffer from information overload, with hundreds if not thousands of sources of information, much of it of poor quality or from thinly veiled commercial sources eager to exploit the desperation of cancer patients.

We need to understand that mass media, whether TV or radio, magazines or newspapers, rarely do a good job at presenting medical information. The constant pressure to simplify messages, and make them "sexier," more uplifting or more controversial, only guarantees superficial and inaccurate treatment of cancer-related issues much of the time. Every patient/consumer ought to consider taking some time to learn how clinical trials are conducted and how to read and evaluate medical research on a basic level. Nothing beats being able to go directly to the research itself. Failing that, identifying the best sources of breast cancer information written for the lay audience becomes essential.

Finally, we need contact with and support from others who have been there. Whether in a face-to-face support group, a conversation with a hotline volunteer, through messages on a bulletin board, chat room or mailing list on the Internet, connection with other women who have been where you are can be deeply healing and informative. The acute sense of isolation and loneliness so many breast cancer patients feel is eased by the knowledge that there are many others out there, eager to reach out to you.

The worried well

Let me offer an important caveat, however. I don't claim to speak for the majority of women who have had breast cancer. It's quite obvious that not everyone feels better with more open discussion, access to information, and contact with other patients. It is what I needed, but it may not be what you need—or what your mother or aunt or best friend needs, for that matter. And that's perfectly okay.

Many breast cancer patients say that they find medical information disturbing, and contact with other women who have had breast cancer depressing. They don't see the value of talking about cancer. They are simply not interested in hearing information about recurrence or what "might happen," and in fact will go to some lengths to avoid exposure to this kind of information. Over the years, I've spoken with many women who want no further contact with breast cancer after treatment is over, and who really do seem determined to be "done with it." At times I have envied their seeming capacity to put the experience away and out of their minds.

Open discussion of health related issues is often related to culture and traditions. There are many elderly women and women from minority and ethnic populations where the prevailing social culture simply doesn't encourage open discussion of cancer, active information-seeking or dialogue with health-care providers.

To a large extent, however, the way we react to having had breast cancer appears to be a matter of temperament. Do you find information and facts fundamentally reassuring, and preferable to the unknown, even if there is some scary news? Not everyone feels this way, as I'm sure you realize from the reactions you've gotten from medical caregivers, family members and some other patients. I have long believed that women with breast cancer fall into two broad categories, in this regard.

Psychological theory agrees with me. In an important paper on coping with illness, well-known Canadian psychiatrist Zbigniew Lipowski theorized that there are two modes of cognitive coping with information in illness. He referred to these modes as "minimization," which implies a tendency to habitually play down the personal significance and emotional impact of a stressful event, and "vigilant focusing," a tendency to respond with a high level of attention and concern that may range from purposeful and rational to exaggerated and obsessive.[3]

In my experience, minimizers are the naturally optimistic, pragmatic women who see no need to worry or to learn more about recurrence until and unless they are forced to deal with it. Barbie and Adele, two women whom I interviewed for this book, are excellent examples. They will deal with the future when it happens. Somewhat fatalistic, they are often content to place their faith in a higher power, and are untroubled by the notion of a personal lack of control. They tend to trust their doctor's treatment recommendations, and ask few detailed questions. Once they've recovered from the physical effects of treatment, they seem to be able to return to their pre-cancer lives with relative ease. It's not that they don't suffer physically with breast cancer treatment—as we all do—but for them, when it's over, it's over. They want to forget it and move on, just as their doctors advise them to do. If the cancer comes back, they will deal with it then—and not a moment sooner. They feel little if any need to be prepared.

Beyond a lack of interest in knowing more about the disease, these women often make an active effort to censor or screen information and talk that may be threatening. While they may volunteer to help others dealing with breast cancer, they don't feel themselves to be at personal risk—or they simply don't allow themselves to think about it. For the most part they are able to put these intrusive thoughts out of their minds. These women are generally not interested in meeting with other survivors, especially not in support groups, where in-depth discussion of emotional concerns may seem irrelevant to them. I have tried to incorporate a few of these voices here.

Vigilant focusers, on the other hand, are the information-seekers like myself. We are women who have been shaken to the core by our diagnoses, and who have had to struggle to get our bearings afterwards. We tend to bore or frighten our friends and families by telling them more about cancer than they really want to know, especially in the early months after diagnosis. While minimizers screen out information, vigilant focusers welcome and thrive on information and often go to great lengths to seek it out. Knowledge gives us some semblance of the sense of control we feel that we've lost. Knowing a lot about our disease, while not without its pitfalls, actually helps us to cope. In fact, in the absence of information, we often find ourselves imagining the worst. The reality, however grim, usually seems preferable to our feared fantasies about it. Our imaginations are, if anything, overactive.

We are the women who read the books, follow the research, search the Internet, join support groups and organizations, seek out the company of other survivors, and become breast cancer advocates. We are the women whom breast cancer touches most deeply, in a variety of ways—not all them negative, by any means.

The median age for breast cancer in the United States is 63, meaning that half of women diagnosed are older, and half younger. For the most part, I believe we represent the younger half, diagnosed in our thirties, forties, fifties and early sixties. Veterans or inheritors of the women's health movement, we cultivate a collaborative relationship with our doctors, in which our many questions and ideas will be welcome.

Most of the voices in this book come from this latter group, but they are often acutely aware of the minimizers around them, as breast cancer patient Deborah states clearly.

> *I work with someone who was diagnosed with breast cancer the same day as I was. She and I had the very same surgery, the very same hour of the same day in different hospitals of the city. We couldn't be more different in our approach to breast cancer. She knows very little about her breast cancer. She doesn't know what kind it is or any of the pathology of it. I'm not even sure she knows if her nodes were involved or if so how many. The day before our surgeries she said to me, "Well, I'm going to tell people tomorrow that this is the start of my cancer-free life." I didn't know what to say. She is done with treatments and from her comments in the last few months she feels very confidant that it's over, that she's cured.*

For the most part, I don't believe that we choose which of these groups we will belong to—although a negative experience with health care or a high-risk diagnosis can at least temporarily radicalize a minimizer and turn her into a vigilant focuser. Conversely, an unsupportive environment can silence a vigilant focuser, and make her feel her concerns are not welcome. Fundamentally, however, what kind of temperament we have is determined by our upbringing and early influences, and probably by our biology.

While I envy the minimizers their fundamentally resilient, optimistic personalities, my allegiance is with the latter group, the "worried well," the women like me. If this describes you, you are my ideal reader, and it's my hope that you'll find lots of common ground, reassurance and information in this book.

CHAPTER 2

Treatment's Over: Now What?

AFTER TREATMENT ENDS, well-meaning friends, family, even trusted medical providers, tend to offer the same familiar advice: that it's time now to focus on family and work again, and get back to life as it was.

As if it were that easy. As if it were possible to explain to anyone who hasn't been changed by a life-threatening illness why that goal may be naïve and unattainable—and probably undesirable, at least for the moment.

You're familiar with the scenario. Your hair is growing in. You don't have to wear your wig anymore. People are telling you they like this smart new boyish look. They're saying things like: "I knew you would beat this thing!" and "Now things can get back to normal."

Would that it were so. If all women who had breast cancer were able to get back to normal after their treatment, healed and ready to go on with their lives, there'd be no need for a book like this. Breast cancer patients would leave their support groups on the last day of their treatment. But the fact of the matter is that many of us find ourselves profoundly changed by our diagnosis and struggling to come to terms with what has happened to us.

We still have questions that remain unanswered, and fears that keep us up at night. Even after hair and fingernails grow back, and reconstructive surgery has been completed, we may still be feeling emotionally fragile. Our bodies and our psyches are different than they were, and we need time, sometimes lots of time, to make sense of the changes and what they mean to us.

This chapter explores the complex feelings women have after completing their treatment for breast cancer, whether it's the end of chemotherapy, the end of five years of tamoxifen, or the completion of reconstructive surgery.

A sense of relief

When treatment ends, the sense of physical compromise that began with diagnosis can begin to resolve, at last. This is especially true when chemotherapy is over, and the toxic chemicals are no longer being pumped into your body. A friend of mine vividly compared recovery from chemotherapy to taking off successive layers of dirty overcoats.

Gradually, the nausea fades and energy returns. Hair begins to grow back, and the wigs, hats and scarves you've been wearing can go back in the drawer—or into the garbage, for you may never be able to bring yourself to wear them again. Surgical scars are beginning to fade. Radiation burns have healed.

In primary breast cancer, it's the treatments, not the disease, that make you sick. So an end to the treatments can feel like a big step down the road toward feeling well again. Of course, women at low risk of recurrence may never have adjuvant treatment, so for them, the end of treatment is signaled by healing from surgery, or completing a course of radiation. Women with pre-invasive cancer or DCIS may finish their treatment with such a good prognosis that recurrence, while still possible, is not much on their minds.

Even for women with a considerable risk for recurrence, there may be a sense of great relief that treatment is over. Mostly, what Francine remembers is being "too exhausted to feel much of anything."

> *The thing I remember most is just being glad that every day I felt better, and that I would keep on feeling better instead of having to undergo another round of chemo and feel worse again. I was very glad to be alive and finally able to eat something. I realized that the meaning of life was food, that life without eating wasn't worth living. Eight months without being able to eat much of anything had been pretty miserable. I was just relieved that it was over. I have a vivid memory of having a bottle of Guinness on February 2nd or 3rd. Nothing ever tasted better. So for me there weren't any mixed emotions.*

Nor were there mixed emotions for Adele.

> *I was glad it was over but it wasn't all that bad. I just got so tired. I worked throughout and think that helped me.*

During her chemo, Adele had found a role model in one of her caregivers, a nurse who was bald and didn't wear a wig.

> *She was beautiful and held her head up and it occurred to me that there was no reason for her not to do so. I figured if she could do it, I could. It worked for me.*

After her treatment ended, Ann threw herself full force into advocacy work, serving on the board of a local cancer support organization.

> When diagnosed, I wasn't working. The combination of not working and the illness was a bit much. Lots of anger. After treatment, I felt relieved. Treatment had lasted nine months from start to finish. Because my tumor (8 cm × 7 cm) had responded so positively to the initial chemo and had reduced significantly prior to surgery, I started looking for small pleasures…like getting my hair back, and then taking on larger challenges like getting a job.

For some, like Debbie, a realistic and pragmatic assessment of their situation seems to come more readily, making the transition into the post-treatment world that much easier.

> I figured—okay, we've given it our best shot. There's no benefit to chemo-forever. Plus, I really do not enjoy medical encounters in any way—I do not like the "feel" of being a patient, so I was very glad to be done with that role. Yes, I had fear, but ending chemo did not affect it either way. By then, I had fully realized the uncertainty, and did not feel strongly that treatment was going to save me (nor that it wouldn't). I saw chemo as one more way to gain an edge. I saw my salvation in the roll of those dice, largely beyond human control. Yet I willingly and with hope availed myself of every treatment available, believing in what the medical community had to offer, but not expecting guarantees.

The unknown companion

When they are first diagnosed, most women believe in the usual breast cancer myths: Medicine has definitive answers. Breast cancer can be cured. If you make it past five years, you're okay. People rarely die of this disease anymore.

It can hurt to find out the truth. For me, the crisis of breast cancer was more than physical, more than emotional—it was also a crisis of belief. It shocked me to discover how much was still unknown about this disease. Treatment choices felt more like guesses, based on imperfect information. The statistics on recurrence and mortality were chilling. And no doctor could give me the assurance I longed for, that I was cured. As I approached the end of treatment, the hard realization dawned that I'd be living with uncertainty for a long, long time. Some remnant, nagging fear of recurrence would be with me for the rest of my life.

My new companion was the unknown. I'd just have to find a way to live with it. It came with the territory.

What will protect me now?

Clearly, the end of treatment marks a transition, not a closure.

For many women, especially those at higher risk of recurrence, breast cancer remains an intimate and ongoing concern, although its presence in awareness will eventually fade with time, if there is no recurrence. The disease has left its evidence written on the book of our bodies, in all the small and large ways that keep it a daily presence in consciousness in these early months and years. Breast cancer confronts us in the mirror each day, affects how we feel in our bodies, appears in our dreams, and ambushes us with tears and irritability as we approach scheduled oncology visits.

Martha had not missed a day's work during her chemotherapy. She was proud of that. Just before her final treatment, she began planning a "No Mo' Chemo" party to thank everyone who had helped her. But something was wrong.

> I started first with crying jags. Crying for no reason I could pinpoint. I began to realize I was dreading the end of chemo in the midst of planning this huge celebration.

Familiar sentiments to me, and to many other breast cancer survivors.

My last treatment was administered Thanksgiving week, 1989. Leaving the oncologist's office that day, I was glad that chemo was over, but also strangely unsettled and apprehensive. I didn't know then what I know now—that ambivalent emotional responses to the end of treatment are quite normal, even commonplace.

At first, it may seem inconceivable that any woman with breast cancer would dread ending a series of chemotherapy treatments that made her bald and sick. Yet these feelings are common. As with everything else, women with breast cancer react to the end of their chemotherapy in a variety of ways.

By far, my strongest fear was that now, with adjuvant treatment over, nothing stood between me and the threat of recurrence. After some initial fear, I'd actually welcomed the chemotherapy, tolerating its side effects by believing that the poisons circulating in my bloodstream had the power to mop up any cancer cells left after surgery. The chemo made me feel safer. Despite the oncologist's reassurances that the benefit afforded by cancer treatments lasts long after the treatment ends, I couldn't shake the feeling I'd been cut adrift. In this fear, as in the others, I was not alone.

Martha describes her feelings at the end of her treatment.

> *I was scared to stop the chemo. While in treatment I was doing something to fight the cancer. I was afraid of what would happen once treatment stopped. To me, I wasn't fighting the cancer. Chemo was. I depended so much on my oncologist. The thought of being released from his care, to go three months without him telling me how well I was doing…what was I going to do? How was I going to face the fear, the what ifs? I found myself sinking.*

Stopping active treatment frightened Deborah, too.

> *I felt that the chemo drugs were protecting me by not allowing breast cancer cells to duplicate and reproduce in my system. From the day of diagnosis I had this incredible fear that there were little undetectable pockets of breast cancer cells throughout my body. I hated that image but I couldn't stop my mind's eye from seeing it. By ending the chemo I felt that I was leaving that security (whether it be real or imagined, accurate or inaccurate) and those stray cells and pockets of cancer would start to grow again.*

With the end of chemo can come the first realization that breast cancer may not be over, as a presence in a woman's life. Those were Maria B's feelings.

> *I thought I'd feel like I'd come to the end of a long dark tunnel, and would celebrate emerging when I finished chemo—but all I saw was more long dark*

> tunnel ahead. I realized then that this cancer stuff
> would be with me for the rest of my life—radiation
> treatments were coming, and then there would be check
> ups, scans, alarms, other biopsies, etc—whether or not
> I still had cancer because it was impossible to know if
> I did or not.

Stopping adjuvant hormonal treatment after five years can also be disconcerting. Despite research that shows that tamoxifen's efficacy lasts far beyond this treatment period, patients can feel exposed and vulnerable at this time. They often feel that the ongoing treatment has been protecting them from recurrence. After his tamoxifen treatment was completed, Bill, a male breast cancer patient, wrote to the Breast-Cancer Mailing List to ask if anyone knew of another drug he could take that could shield him from recurrence now.

> I am having some qualms about stopping tamoxifen
> cold turkey. My oncologist said that stopping treatment
> after five years is the current standard of care and
> medically this is what he would recommend.

Bill looked into taking another kind of hormonal drug, but found out there was no research to indicate that it would help. But he didn't feel comfortable with doing nothing.

> I wanted to scream at the doctor, "TELL ME WHAT
> TO DO!" but that is not his role. I am more frustrated
> and worried about the decision I have to make than
> when I was first diagnosed. When I was first diagnosed
> it was pretty easy. Based on my biopsy it was evident
> that a mastectomy, chemo, and radiation was the way
> to go. Maybe I was too ignorant or in an emotional
> daze at the time, but the decisions then seemed to be
> a no-brainer. Now I don't know what to do.

After the crisis

Most anyone can gear up for a crisis. The shock and grief of diagnosis, the confusing treatment options and second opinions, the realities of surgery, chemotherapy and radiation—all of this unfolds so rapidly, carrying us along with little time to make sense of it all. The need to rise to the occasion often translates to a sort of putting-one-foot-in-front-of-the-other stoicism. We learn to get through it, to face fears, to find strengths we hadn't known were there.

From the time of my diagnosis, through surgery and the six months of my own chemotherapy, I'd been in a crisis mentality, psyching myself up for the onslaught of surgery, chemo, and reconstruction.

Then, all of a sudden—nothing. It was over.

I was left with an echoing silence when the oncologist turned me loose, holding nothing but an appointment slip three months hence. Three months! It seemed like forever.

The loss of support from their medical team often leaves patients feeling a bit bereft, as Maria W found.

> Initially I was thrilled to be finished! Within weeks, however, I was about as low as I'd ever been. Suddenly, I had no more appointments for as much as a month at a time! I still looked the part because of no hair, still felt the part because of no energy, but I wasn't getting the frequent support from my nurses and doctors. For eight months my disease had been getting attention from so many, and now I was almost on my own. It was scary and I was depressed.

With inflammatory breast cancer, Bonnie had undergone intensive chemo, radiation and a bone marrow transplant. Initially, she says, she described herself as "euphoric" on her release from the transplant unit after 25 days there. But the feelings didn't last.

> *The most difficult time for me was after all my treatment was over. I had spent many hours with doctors and nurses for many months. Once I was healthy enough to move to three-month appointments, I missed their reassurance and support. It took a while for me to regain my independence and feel secure without their constant encouragement.*

Feeling alone

After finishing chemotherapy, many women miss the camaraderie of the treatment room, or of the hospital-based support groups they may have joined during treatment. Oncology nurses and other patients have provided much-needed companionship and reassurance.

For Diane, the sense of confronting this threat together with other women turned out to be more important than she had realized.

> *I attended my last CMF treatment four years ago with four friends—we'd all traveled the same route together. Before the injections we were all laughing and joking, saying how great it all was that we'd finished. After the infusions we all sat and looked at one another, almost too worn out to breathe. None of us wanted anything to eat, none of us could think of anything to say, and none of us wanted to be the first to get up and walk out of the chemo suite. In the end, of course, we all did. I cried my way to my car, cried all the way home, and all that evening and most of the night. My friends all phoned up that evening and said how*

pleased they were that it was over, but I couldn't even
take the calls. My husband spoke to them all. I think
that the day treatment finished was the loneliest in my
life. I was out there on my own, I felt, for the first time.

Others sometimes can compound the loneliness, without meaning to. Friends, family members, husbands and partners— most of the people in our lives are more than ready for this breast cancer ordeal to be over. And who can blame them? The spoken or unspoken message from those who have supported us is often: "It's time to get on with your life."

During the six months of my own chemotherapy, my friends and family stayed closed by, letting me know in large and small ways that they cared. People often told me how courageous I was, that I was coping so well. But I could sense toward the end how ready they were for me to move on.

"You look great!" friends would say enthusiastically when they saw me. "Thanks," I'd learned to respond, "I feel fine."

At first, I'd tried giving accurate bulletins to friends who asked how I was, and some who didn't. But after a few months, my litany of complaints had become tiresome, even to me. Yet the cancer was still very much on my mind.

When I began talking with other women who'd had breast cancer, I discovered that I was far from alone in my perception that others didn't want to know how I really felt. The reactions of others—or rather, their lack of reaction—turned out to be a common concern. Suzanne recounted a typical situation.

What I don't know how to cope with is the effect of
my living with breast cancer on some of those closest to
me. This year when I planned to walk for the second
time in the Race for the Cure, my sister was "too busy"

to join me as planned. She offered to make a pledge,
but also subtly suggested that I might have a more fun
day doing something else.

Friends or family members may discourage what they believe to be an unhealthy continuing "preoccupation" with issues related to breast cancer.

Suzanne spoke of this with some bitterness.

Few of my loved ones ask me how I'm doing now
that treatment is over, and I must admit to being
reluctant to bring up the topic myself. There is this
sense that it is over and done with—that I have been
a "brave girl" (whatever that means), but it's all over.
That the subject is closed.

Letting down

After the long siege of diagnosis and treatment has passed, a period of "letting down" can occur. While not universal by any means, difficulty during this period of time is very common.

It may be especially apparent in women who have felt the need to "tough it out" during their treatment, determined to put on a brave face and keep their lives as normal as possible for their families. Some are determined never to reveal their cancer diagnosis or treatment to colleagues at work, or to acquaintances, and take pride in being able to conceal their illness. These heroic efforts can take a big toll.

When treatment is finally over, and it is "safe" to let it out, such a woman can feel overwhelmed by the outpouring of emotions she has been holding in. Later, she can become depressed and anxious as she realizes the extent to which uncertainty has taken up residence in her life.

Looking back at my own reaction, I can see this process clearly at work. The grief I'd been too afraid and too numb to feel settled heavily around me. My ongoing anxieties reached a crescendo at the time of each follow-up visit to my oncologist. I couldn't help wondering if there was something wrong with me. Subsequently, I learned from other women I met that this is a time when we are particularly vulnerable to emotions we may have suppressed during treatment. And that I was far from alone in fearing that something was wrong with me.

Marjorie found the whole experience devastating.

> I have always taken challenges and trials in stride
> and I've had many in my life, but I was face down in
> the dirt on this one. People kept telling me how
> inspirational and brave I was and I felt like a fraud.
> I wasn't brave and I was questioning my faith.

A delayed or missed diagnosis can create a special sense of bitterness and despair, as Barbara discovered when the full impact of her invasive recurrence following DCIS finally hit her.

> I didn't really put the whole mess together and let it
> sink in until I was done with the chemo. I became
> deeply depressed, panic-stricken and suicidal, but this
> was more because I realized the cancer I had had been
> avoidable. When I thought I was just dealing with life,
> I was okay. It was when I realized that the doctors I'd
> been going to could have truly cured me, just by
> explaining things better to me, I couldn't take it.

For Marjorie and her husband, seeking professional help made a real difference.

> We sought counseling because I found myself crying
> at almost anything.. I was full of anger and remorse
> over this sad turn of events in my life. I had always

known cancer was a possibility and had been very
diligent since both my parents died of cancer. I didn't
know how to proceed with so much uncertainty
surrounding me.

Not every aspect of this letting down is related to fear of recurrence, of course. At the end of chemotherapy, most women are simply sick and tired of feeling sick and tired. Many of the emotions women feel at this time are tied up with physical changes, especially the changes of chemotherapy induced menopause or hormonal treatments, and, of course, the scars and losses of breast surgery.

For women who've had reconstructive surgery, a major let-down in the post-treatment experience can occur if there are less than satisfactory final results, after the months of anticipation and surgeries. Caroline captured those feelings well.

I'm grieving for my own soft, wobbly, small,
individual breasts all over again. Three years of
breastfeeding, 51 years old, they were nothing to write
home about. But I miss them dreadfully.

This seems to be the time, at last, when you have to
put a brave face on things and tell everyone how
pleased you are with your new boobs. That's what I'm
doing, anyway. My body has a major image problem
these days, and I'm not going to contribute to
undermining it in public in any way. I've got a PR job
ahead of me.

My reconstructed breasts look as though they belong
to a female nude produced by a fourth-rate sculptor
who's never actually seen a woman naked. They are
generic lumps. I know I'll get round to appreciating
them some time down the track. I'll probably even be

polite about them to my surgeon tomorrow! Probably
I made the right decision in going for reconstruction
(I'm not sure about this—I very much admire the
women who go without—and I think if I'd had longer
to think about the decision I might at least have
postponed reconstruction.) But right now I feel like I've
got a pair of prostheses off the shelf, grafted onto my
chest. Which, come to think of it, I have.

With the end of treatment, breast cancer patients reach a major milestone along the long strange journey that is breast cancer. While the world outside may see this juncture as a cause for celebration, for us, the experience is often decidedly mixed.

The week after my last chemotherapy treatment, my husband's family gathered for Thanksgiving dinner. There was little to be thankful for that year. One of my brothers-in-law had died at 53 of esophageal cancer not two months before. My father-in-law stood and tearfully raised his glass in a tribute to his son Robert and other members of the family who'd died of cancer in recent years. Queasily moving the turkey and stuffing around on my plate, I was keeping my head down and trying not to cry, when my father-in-law, still standing, turned to me and wished me well.

It is always that bittersweet Thanksgiving day that comes to mind, when I think of the end of my treatment.

CHAPTER 3

Cure and Survivor: Two Troubling Words

"CURE" AND "SURVIVOR" are arguably two of the most widely used—yet misunderstood—words used in talking about breast cancer. Since breast cancer can recur after many years, absolute certainty of cure is beyond reach, for most breast cancer patients. Women have various responses to acquiring the title of breast cancer survivor, given that reality. The experience of uncertainty is a continuing thread. As Maria B dryly put it, "Having a diagnosis of cancer seems to require a very large tolerance for ambiguity."

In this chapter, we explore what the concept of cure means to patients, to statisticians and researchers, and to physicians. What do you say when someone asks if you are cured? How is "cure" used by the media and cancer organizations? What complex meanings are embodied in the term, "survivor"?

The "C" word

Once upon a time, cancer was referred to, in hushed tones, as the "C" word. Now we're past such euphemisms. But despite this new openness, for many breast cancer survivors there is a new "C" word—cure—spoken with an edge of irony and even bitterness, when uttered at all.

The fact is, cure is a word that media loves to use and the public loves to hear. It's upbeat, implying victory over a life experience fraught with fear, a comforting antidote to the anxieties women feel about this dread disease. Its calming influence encourages women examine their breasts and get mammograms, or so the authorities on early detection would have us believe. It also helps breast cancer patients accept and justify the difficult treatments they are told they must undergo.

But over-optimistic media coverage about cure makes many breast cancer survivors angry. "Breast cancer has a very high cure rate, with 97 percent of women surviving for five years if the cancer is diagnosed early," trumpeted website Yahoo! Health, in a webpage devoted to Breast Cancer Awareness Month.

The five-year survival statistic is accurate but misleading. Five-year survival is not equivalent to cure. The 97 percent figure includes not only those whose cancer has not recurred, but those whose cancer has and are still alive. It also includes those whose cancer may still recur but whose possible recurrences are delayed by chemotherapy and the anti-estrogen drug tamoxifen. Breast cancer tends to be slow-growing and better treatments have extended life for metastatic patients. So, while 75 percent of recurrences happen within five years, fully one quarter of all recurrences occur after the five-year period. Furthermore, up to 35 percent of women with metastatic breast cancer now live five or more years following recurrence. So, as breast cancer outcomes improve over time, short-term statistics are becoming less meaningful.

What is meant by the word "cure"

What cure means depends upon who's using the word, and for what purpose. To statisticians, it means one thing, to doctors another, and to breast cancer activists and patients, something else again.

With no entry between "curare" and "curettage," my medical dictionary is no help, while trusty Webster's weighs in by saying that cure "specifically suggests the elimination of a disease." This is how I think of the word. When we are cured of bronchitis, with an antibiotic, we mean it is gone for good. If we get sick again, it's a new episode of illness. In daily speech, cure often also has a sense of the absolute and forever attached to it.

The medical literature on breast cancer uses the term only rarely, preferring measurable data to unfounded speculation about the future. The highly regarded (and quite weighty!) medical text on breast cancer that graces my bookshelf indexes the word cure only once, referring to it with this cryptic statement: "Many patients never develop distant metastases and these may be considered cured."

But considered by whom, and at what point in time? When Esther pressed her doctor to say whether she was cured, he presented the current state of medical knowledge (or lack thereof) with a humorous twist.

> *If, when you are 99 years old, you die of a heart attack, you were cured. If, when you are 99 years old, you die of cancer, you were in remission.*

Not every doctor is as honest with patients about the vagaries of prognosis. Whether this approach derives from a need to reassure a frightened patient, or is simply a throwback to an earlier, paternalistic era in medicine, women can and do feel betrayed when doctors tell them they are cured, and their breast cancer comes back anyway.

Doreen, who developed metastatic disease in her bones, after an initial breast cancer diagnosis fifteen years earlier, was still angry at her doctors for their misleading initial prognosis.

> *I feel cheated. I shouldn't have been told that I was cured. It was devastating when I realized what had been happening. I would have planned my life differently.*

What most women I've spoken with seem to want from their doctors is the truth, presented with sensitivity, and with a sense of the limitations of prognosis. If we don't know, we don't know. We can handle that. But we need to feel our doctors will level with us. Julie's response was typical of the women I asked.

> *I like hope. But I prefer the truth to false hope. So please, no "cure" for me, until you can guarantee it in writing.*

Some oncologists shade their advice more subtly, and perhaps more wisely, suggesting that patients should "consider" themselves cured as an antidote to the perpetual anxiety and vigilance of living with the fear of recurrence.

After her treatment, Sara M's doctor told her:

> *"You've got to believe you are cured." Not "You are cured." That was okay by me. Oh I didn't believe it then of course... and still don't, really. But I'm closer than two years ago, for sure. If I do*

> *have a recurrence, I will deal with it as and when.*
> *Meanwhile, in the absence of any guarantees,*
> *hoping that I am truly cured is okay for now.*

The reasoning behind this kind of advice appears to be that living with a state of uncertainty is either impossible or intolerable. For obvious reasons, those, like Sara, with very early stage disease may find this mental discipline easier.

But as patients begin to comprehend the ambiguity and uncertainty surrounding their disease, and confront mortality for what is, perhaps, the first time in their lives, they often experience a certain loss of innocence. Jan spoke for many, when she said:

> *At diagnosis I felt so out of control. But then I*
> *finally realized that I had never really had control.*
> *I was blissfully ignorant prior to breast cancer and*
> *felt like nothing could ever happen to me.*

You may find that hearing other breast cancer patients share their stories and share information is disillusioning for you. Learning about the disease is not without emotional risks. The trade-off for getting information and support with other survivors is often a poignant one. You may end up exchanging isolation for anxiety; innocence for knowledge.

Am I cured?

Many women believe they are cured of their breast cancer after their treatment is over. They may be only dimly aware that they still run a risk of recurrence. Some, like Sara, are advised that believing they are cured is their best way to cope. Others feel that even entertaining this positive belief is a cop-out, a form of avoidance.

This can be a touchy topic for women who've had breast cancer, when they get together to talk, as Sharon M found out.

> I remember a time in the past when we had this discussion here on the list, and the thread took on the subject line: "Pretending you're cured" to which my response was "What's wrong with that?" I still feel that way.

Sharon described her initial diagnosis and eight-year remission prior to her recurrence.

> After that, I was quite happy to turn my back on breast cancer, leave it behind me, and thankfully consider myself "cured." Sure, I got nervous at check-up time, but the longer I went without recurrence, the more confident I became. Some people would consider such behavior the equivalent of burying my head in the sand or denying reality. But I think my behavior, at least for me, was very healthy. I learned from my "close call" to appreciate my friends and family all the more, and I learned to do those things that were important to me and to say no to those that were not.

Bonnie found herself agreeing with Sharon M.

> I work hard at living my life as if I will be alive for the foreseeable future. I choose (and it is an often difficult choice) not to die before I die. So if you meet me you will most often find me upbeat and optimistic.

A recent scare had made Bonnie realize she would live the rest of her life "on a rickety bridge."

And then the bone biopsy came back negative.
I thought about how my conversation with my
doctor made it perfectly clear that I did not have
the luxury of believing that I would live a long
time—that, in fact, I could "light up the bone scan"
in a couple of years and be on a track for death. So
now I know (as if I didn't know before). And
nothing has changed. I thought about this and went
back to being my old, upbeat self.

For these two women, thinking of themselves as being cured became a strategy for coping, one that they share with many other breast cancer patients—but by no means all.

If you want to stimulate controversy among women diagnosed with breast cancer, just utter the word "cure."

Deborah, for example, had a very different perception.

To me cured means that every cell of the cancer
is totally out of my body. No one will ever be able
to tell me that with certainty. I will never know
whether every cell is gone or if some cells are there
dividing. And somehow I feel that the cancer is not
all out. It's frightening and sobering. But I think it's
more realistic to think this way than the other way.

John's views about cure were clearly informed by the metastatic disease his wife was suffering.

When so many have recurrences, I don't think
the word "cure" is honest. Some survive, in some
the cancer stays asleep. When I think of "cure",
I think of the Salk vaccine and polio. I think of
disease I know only from reading history books.
And I look forward to the time, when someone

> *much younger than I asks if I remember when*
> *people got cancer.*

When Ellen's tumor markers became elevated, she was not surprised.

> *I never thought of myself as cured, even after*
> *eight years. I know breast cancer too well. Because*
> *my tumor involved so many nodes and had invaded*
> *the walls of several, I doubted that all of the cells*
> *could have been killed even by the heroic*
> *chemotherapy used. I've been waiting for the other*
> *shoe to drop.*

Slogans and statistics

The word cure is often used as a reminder of what advocates are working for, as a rallying cry, a slogan. But when we speak of a cure for breast cancer, it's a distantly glimpsed ultimate objective—an artificially unified goal, held in contrast to increasingly complex research realities. While some organizations race for the cure, drive for the cure, even shop for the cure, other organizations, it must be said, carefully avoid the "C" word. Instead they declare as a goal "eradicating" breast cancer, a word whose first meaning is to "tear out by the roots," implying a concern with prevention as well as treatment, and embracing a goal that doesn't inaccurately imply a single method or magic bullet.

Nevertheless, statistically speaking, it seems clear that breast cancer can indeed be cured, if by cure one means that many patients treated for the disease live without recurrence for several decades, and eventually die of other causes.

This was not always the perception. Early studies on the natural history of breast cancer led to the belief that for the rest of their lives, a percentage of women who'd once had breast cancer would continue to recur and ultimately die from the disease.

As recently as 1991, a large Italian study looking back at the history of more than five thousand breast cancer patients found "evidence of a persistent excess mortality"—an increased death rate from breast cancer—"even after long-term follow-up" of twenty years. The authors concluded that their findings had "provided no evidence of a 'clinical' cure for breast cancer patients." Even node-negative disease—breast cancer that had not spread outside the breast at the time of diagnosis—the authors suggested, should be thought of as "a slow-growing metastatic disease."[1]

However, a longer-term University of Chicago study published in 1999 in the *Journal of the National Cancer Institute* found that most recurrences happened within ten years of diagnosis, and were very rare after twenty years. After this length of time, the death rates matched those of the rest of the population, the authors concluded.[2]

A population-based study that looked at all breast cancer cases from a single urban area in Finland from 1945 to 1965 found no excess of breast cancer deaths after 27 years, excluding patients who developed breast cancer in the other breast.[3]

A similar Dutch study concluded that, "Patients who survive for 19 years may be considered cured." And finally, a statistical analysis conducted on survival data for 13,000 women with breast cancer in Utah over a 30-year period concluded that "cure is a possible outcome of breast cancer treatment."[4]

The best overall statistics on long-term survival we have in the United States are from the Surveillance, Epidemiology, and End Results (SEER) Program of the National Cancer Institute (NCI), which is based on eleven representative cancer registries around the United States that include 14 percent of the entire U.S. population.[5] The NCI includes particular registries because of the quality of their data, and the fact that their communities reflect overall US demographics. These cancer registries collect data on patient demographics, primary tumor sites, stage at diagnosis, among other information. Established in 1973, since 1976, SEER has been tracking cancer mortality, as well as incidence.

According to SEER data, for those diagnosed with breast cancer in 1976, relative mortality from the disease was 49.7 percent. That means a little more than half of patients treated in 1976 have survived their breast cancer—at least until 1999, the last year for which figures are available. This figure is adjusted to account for other causes of death. But with recent advances in treatment and with earlier diagnosis, the clinical cure rate is almost certainly much higher now for women diagnosed today, as we will see in Chapter 5, *Everything You Wanted to Know About Recurrence*. Indeed, later SEER data clearly reflect significant improvement in survival rates.

No evidence of disease (NED)

Even though the survival rates are improving, the reality is we live with uncertainty, and cure is too absolute a word. It implies a confidence we will never possess again, a recapturing of innocence lost. For most of us, cure implies permanence and completion: when you're cured of an illness, it's done, you're restored to your former state of health.

As we've already discussed, even if breast cancer never recurs, this disease has a way of leaving us changed psychologically, emotionally and physically. Scar tissue, disfigurement, lymphedema, premature menopause, chemobrain, fatigue, loss of sensation, and other lasting side effects of treatment make it difficult for many of us to think in terms of a cure. So we struggle, instead, for a "new normal."

Suzanne put it this way:

> *My problem with the word "cure" is this: what does it mean to me and my way of coping with a potentially life threatening and certainly life altering disease? Can I ever relax, and say to myself, "Well I am surely going to die some day, but it won't be from breast cancer—whew!" For me the word cure is a paradox, full of contradictions.*
>
> *I will never be the same again. Never fully well (or enjoying the illusion of it), never able to completely relax. For you see, the most important definition of 'cured' for me would be to be able to assume the best, that I am well, that it won't happen again.*

So what word should those of us who have completed treatment with no sign of recurrence use to describe our state of being? Do we have breast cancer, or did we have it? Present tense or past? Saying we're in remission is just the fatalistic flip-side of the cure coin, implying that somewhere within us the cancer is dormant or growing but still undetected. We can't know that, either.

Many of us have chosen to label our current status just as the doctors do: N.E.D. The initials stand for "no evidence of disease," meaning that breast cancer may be there, lurking about, or it may not. It's beyond the ability of current medical science to measure that. It's what we know now. It's all that we know, and that's good enough. It has to be.

In a world of pink ribbons and supposed 97 percent cure rates, we choose uncertainty. We choose truth.

Survivor

The term "survivor" inspires almost as much discussion and diversity of opinion as the word "cure" does among women who've had breast cancer. While I use the term more easily now to describe myself, in the early years after my diagnosis, I was suspicious of it, as if I was tempting fate.

When I looked it up in the dictionary, I discovered that a survivor was one who exists longer than another, one who outlives. So, not only did the term "survivor"—like "cure"—lay claim an essentially unknowable outcome, but it also seemed to divide breast cancer patients into two groups: those who lived and those who died of the disease. Using it felt disloyal to the women from my support group who had died, and to the tens of thousands of others who die each year.

For Debbie, the term felt judgmental.

> I don't like the word "survivor." To me, it implies something about those who have not survived. The survivors are stronger, somehow more worthy — they survived not because of the roll of the dice in the crapshoot, but because they "fought harder," or had a "better attitude," or a "stronger will." This leaves those who died in the "weak and wimpy" category, by default. Some thank God for blessing them with survival—which again by default, means God frowned upon, or found unworthy, those who did not survive. That bothers me, a lot. I know strong, brave souls who have died of cancer.
>
> It makes me very uncomfortable when acquaintances say, "I just knew you were going to beat this—you're so positive, and so strong." I think, "bullshit," but I thank them for their

> *thoughts, knowing they mean well. I prefer the*
> *word "veteran." Or when it fits the context, I say*
> *"I was treated for breast cancer."*

Marjorie also thought of the word "survivor" in terms of military metaphors.

> *There are days when I use the term survivor with*
> *great pride and other days when I dislike it*
> *immensely. It's a weird title but I know it's a label*
> *that fits, like it or not. Anyone who isn't dead is a*
> *survivor, cancer or not. It's like the term "veteran."*
> *War, like cancer, is hell, but you've been there and*
> *so you wear the label. The idea is not letting that*
> *label define your life.*

For Maria W, the distinction was more subtle.

> *"Survivor" can imply having withstood an ordeal.*
> *In that sense, I do not think of myself as a cancer*
> *survivor. I have never had any symptom of cancer*
> *except for a lump. Never any pain, never any*
> *dysfunction, no weakness, no physical losses.*
> *Perhaps I think of myself as a chemo survivor.*
> *Having chemo was the most frightening thing I've*
> *done in my life. It is hard for me to remember that*
> *the chemo effects are from the chemo and not from*
> *the cancer—cancer and chemo go together in my*
> *mind.*

As a psychotherapist, Ellen speculates on the motivations behind the use of the word "survivor."

> *I've been trying for eight years to think of a*
> *better word. I nearly died at birth because of*
> *trauma to my right arm. I survived that, an acute*
> *event. But cancer is a disease process. My sister*

had quadruple bypass surgery, which saved her life,
but we don't call her a "heart surgery survivor."
If I had to choose a way to express being cancer-
free, I would simply say, "I'm cancer free at this
time."

Perhaps the need to use a single word to signify
that one has finished treatment is a symbolic way of
putting an end to the cancer nightmare. We use the
word "survivor" to refer to Holocaust victims.
Cancer patients are not victims; they have an
illness. Cancer is not victimizing anyone. It simply
exists. I believe that choosing a word to signify the
end of treatment is like trying to ward off a curse.
Cancer still has the aura of being dirty, shameful,
disgusting, and needing to be hidden. The use of a
word is like magical thinking to free us of the dirty
devil: thus, survivor.

Over time, however, many women come to embrace the title of
survivor as a badge of courage. Kate, who has been diagnosed
not only with breast cancer, but with ovarian and colon cancer
as well, felt this strongly.

I do think of myself as a survivor, not so much
because I am NED (no evidence of disease), but
because I lived through the diagnosis and treatment
of breast cancer and became stronger and healthier
as a result. I have never felt defeated by the disease,
although there have been some very frightening
times when I thought I was dealing with a
recurrence.

For Kate, taking an active stance has been integral to her sense
of survivorship.

> *I don't think you can live with breast or any*
> *other cancer and remain passive. Survivors do*
> *more than just get "cured," they grab hold and*
> *hang on.*

Being a breast cancer survivor has altered Emma's perspective on aging.

> *I was talking last week to someone I met who*
> *challenged me when I suggested that turning 54*
> *isn't traumatic. She said, "You're not there yet. How*
> *do you know?" I took a breath and said, "I do know.*
> *Two years ago, I was diagnosed with cancer. I used*
> *to dread each year of aging, and now I hope I'll get*
> *to be a really old woman."*

For Bonnie, the word encompassed a triumph of spirit over adversity.

> *To me, a survivor is someone who has endured a*
> *catastrophic life event (such as a devastating*
> *illness, an accident, or a personal loss) and is able*
> *to find purpose and pleasure in the days and years*
> *that follow—despite the memories and the pain.*

The last decade brought a great deal of adversity into Bonnie's life. Her inflammatory breast cancer diagnosis, and subsequent bone marrow transplant was followed by a serious automobile accident that hospitalized her for many months. Somehow, Bonnie was able to emerge with her positive beliefs intact.

> *I'm comfortable with the word survivor—so*
> *much so that my license plate says SAVIVA (which*
> *is how we say survivor in Massachusetts).*

CHAPTER 4

Follow-up Visits and Worrisome Symptoms

IF YOU COULD LOOK INSIDE the minds and hearts of breast cancer patients in the months and years following diagnosis, you would find some common features, bound by a single emotion: anxiety. Worrying is a central part of the post-treatment landscape.

We are worried about recurrence. Oh, it's not all day, every day, of course, but at certain times, when certain events seem inevitably to trigger these fears. We know that breast cancer can come back, even after many years. We worry about how we are ever going to make peace with that uncertainty. And we know that when breast cancer metastasizes, it can rarely be cured. We worry how we would ever be able to cope emotionally if we had a recurrence. Before our routine follow-up appointments, we worry the doctor will find something. Afterwards, we worry about test results, and we worry about not being tested enough. We are afraid that recurrence means painful treatments and imminent death. We worry how our families would manage without us. When a friend or acquaintance has a recurrence, we feel more vulnerable. We wonder if we might be next. We aren't sure what symptoms to look for that would suggest recurrence, so any ache or pain that lasts is worrisome. We prod, poke and obsessively examine the lumps, bumps and painful spots we fear might be "something." We try not to share our worries with our families and friends, either to protect them, or because we're afraid we'll be judged for worrying too much. We feel badly that we haven't been able to "put it behind us" and "get back to normal." And we worry that something is wrong with us, that it's not normal to worry as much as we do.

Our worries are imponderables, grounded in uncertainty. There are no answers. But there is sharing. This chapter takes you on a journey through the landscape of post-treatment worries. Reading about other women's anxieties will help you to feel you aren't alone, that the worries you have are perfectly normal—even inevitable. Expressing those fears, sharing them with others, and even learning to laugh about them in time, all become important steps toward recovery.

Follow-up visits: Anything but routine

Women who have had breast cancer often feel a great deal of apprehension when they return to their oncologist's office for routine follow-up visits, especially during the first year or two. It's not uncommon for women to experience more physical and emotional symptoms in the days preceding these visits, like insomnia and irritability. I certainly did.

I've learned since that my response is not unusual, and that it can last for years. While women learn to cope with these feelings and often value their relationships with their doctors, the feelings of apprehension are still there.

However successfully we manage to deal with the fact that breast cancer may return many years after diagnosis, the anxiety is still there, lurking. What better focus than a scheduled doctor's appointment, especially with the very doctor who provided the initial treatment? We can't help but develop all sorts of disturbing associations, not only with the doctor, but with the treatment rooms, the nurses and receptionist, the waiting room, the building, the street—even the part of town. We may not even be consciously aware of the source of our symptoms. However beautiful Central Park may look, my heart still sinks when I pass the corner of Fifth Avenue and 96th Street in Manhattan. And my oncologist has yet to get a normal blood pressure reading from me, even after fourteen years of follow-up visits.

A year and a half after finishing treatment for her Stage IIA diagnosis, Marjorie felt ambivalent. On the one hand, she was upset about seeing her doctor less frequently. She was also fearful that even when she did, something would be wrong and they wouldn't find it.

> *I was very neurotic when my check ups moved
> to three-month intervals. I had become
> "institutionalized" in a way. When I was no longer
> seeing my oncologist or going to the lab weekly, I
> was very fearful that something vital was going to
> be missed. I'm still fearful that I won't recognize
> something as being abnormal and get to the doctor
> in time—or worse, they'll miss it like the first time
> with my mammogram.*

But as Marjorie got used to the less frequent visits to her oncologist, she noticed a difference in her response.

> *It's beginning to get better and I'm calming down
> as time progresses. Yet, whenever someone I know
> has a recurrence, I begin the battle against fear all
> over again. My doctors have to prove to me I'm*

> *healthy now. Everything has reversed and I no*
> *longer trust my body.*

Diagnosed at Stage IIB, Maria B described her visits to her oncologist this way:

> *At first, I wanted him to tell me the answer—*
> *was I going to live or was cancer going to kill me?*
> *After about two years, I no longer expect him to*
> *answer the unanswerable. I still think about dying*
> *every day—usually every night, but I don't fret*
> *about it too long. I think denial has its uses.*

With only two follow-up visits with her oncologist under her belt, normally stoic Debbie, diagnosed at Stage II, still faced reactions to these routine checkups that she had not anticipated.

> *Returning to that office, recalling, not mentally,*
> *but in a whole-body, uncontrollable-response way,*
> *those first surreal moments of walking through a*
> *door labeled CANCER—so "otherworldly," outside*
> *of anything I ever expected to happen in my*
> *world—those feelings come back strongly, no*
> *matter how composed and together I think I am.*
> *This is somewhat tempered by the fact that I do like*
> *to visit with my oncologist, and see my chemo-*
> *nurse. Once I get through the door, I'm okay.*

Five years after her Stage I diagnosis at age 32 halfway through her first pregnancy, Sharon B said:

> *I don't often feel terrified before appointments*
> *or anything, but yet there are definite anxiety*
> *symptoms that come up for me at those times. I will*
> *be sleepless for a few days or break out in a rash.*
> *It's very annoying!*

Six years after her Stage IIIA diagnosis, Francine was still a bundle of nerves when her checkups roll around.

> I'm always surprised at the degree of anxiety I have about the exam and the results. I've been about the same all along. It just doesn't seem to go away.

Dianne was diagnosed seven years ago with Stage II breast cancer.

> Once my initial treatments were over, I tried to steer clear of the medical community as much as possible. I'm not quite sure what has prompted this response, but I never feel "safe" when I have to see a doctor. Now, a cold always feels more threatening. A sore throat, an ache ... and because I've had breast cancer, if I mention any of the above, they usually want to run some tests.

Nancy S was diagnosed with Stage IIB breast cancer six years ago.

> Over time, I feel less need to be followed closely. I still get frightened at check up time, but I also find that I actually forget to make my follow up appointments until about a month before they are due.

Sometimes anxiety can be tied to a doctor or an institution. Because of her high-risk diagnosis at Stage IIIA, Ellen participated in a clinical trial protocol of an aggressive and debilitating chemotherapy regimen, as well as post-mastectomy radiation. Afterwards, she had a hard time visiting the place where the treatments took place.

> During the protocol period I was intensely anxious. Going through the same corridors and to

the same radiology suite provoked a deja vu, *as if
I still were receiving chemo. Each time I had a chest
x-ray or any other x-ray I would sit waiting for the
result and tell myself "I don't know, I don't know."
This was to prevent myself from thinking the worst.*

*Initially, I was followed every three months by
my doctor. This lasted for five years because I was
on a protocol. I felt safe because of the frequent
visits. When I finished the five-year period, my
doctor said that I could come every six months.
I preferred to come every three months because
I was so anxious.*

When Ellen moved from New York City to the West coast, her
feelings shifted.

*Once away from there I felt much less anxious
and was followed yearly here in California.
Entering my new Cancer Center no longer made
me anxious. I stopped being so vigilant and forgot
about breast cancer most of the time.*

Back in 1996, Bonnie was accustomed to the frequent doctor's
visits that followed her high-dose chemotherapy with stem-cell
transplant for inflammatory breast cancer.

*I'm a worrier by nature, so I'm always
evaluating whether a pain or a bruise or a lump
should be checked out. In recent years, however,
I've come to trust myself more and am much more
comfortable with self-evaluation.*

*Since my transplant, I have had a skin biopsy, a
lumpectomy, a rib biopsy and an MRI to rule out
recurrence, so my life isn't exactly a smooth ride,*

> *but I do okay and as I undergo more and more of*
> *these tests, I become less fearful of the future.*

Three years later, Bonnie described how it had felt to be "graduating" to seeing her oncologist only every three months.

> *I appreciate the careful monitoring but still cope*
> *with the fears that these tests and office visits*
> *engender. Yesterday, my first three-monther, my*
> *oncologist felt my shoulder blades and said,*
> *"My God, you are so tense!" I responded, "What*
> *do you expect? I am terrified to be here."*

Bonnie couldn't help wondering how this normally perceptive oncologist who knew her so well could be unaware of how stressful these office visits were.

> *This is a woman who is dedicated to her job, lost*
> *her mom to breast cancer, and is very sensitive to*
> *all of us. When I am half naked on that examining*
> *table and this young physician is moving her fingers*
> *over my body with the intensity and concentration*
> *of a rocket scientist, I am not calm. I am watching*
> *her eyes and waiting for those fingers to stop and*
> *wondering what she will ask me about or make an*
> *appointment for.*

Some of us have to survive

All of the women I know who've had breast cancer—if only by virtue of my knowing them—know at least one other person else with the disease. Most of them know many more, in their families, their communities, their support groups and organizations, online and in "real life." In the fourteen years since my own diagnosis, doing the work that I do, I've met literally thousands of other women with breast cancer, women struggling at every stage along a complicated continuum, from terror stricken on the day of diagnosis to lying in hospice care—and many like the lovely older woman who approached me at a book signing in California just three weeks after my surgery, to whisper in my ear that she'd had her mastectomy 25 years ago, and was just fine.

When I joined a support group midway through my chemotherapy, I was so exhilarated at this wonderful opportunity to air my feelings, and find out that they weren't so abnormal, after all, that I didn't stop to think about what might happen years down the line, if we stayed close. As it turns out, we have stayed very close. In the fourteen years that we've been friends, we've shared innumerable feelings, stories, laughter and tears. But we've also shared what every support group that stays in touch with one another shares—recurrences and deaths. Of the nine women who formed my support group, five are still meeting with some regularity, and three of us have died of breast cancer.

More of our story appears in Chapter 7, *The People in Your Life,* but some discussion belongs in this chapter as well. There is no doubt that a major source of anxiety about recurrence comes from direct exposure to women we know—women like us—who have their cancer recur, and who ultimately die of the disease. It's one thing to know this in the abstract, quite another to lose a friend or a member of your own support group.

For some, the difficulties soon outweigh the benefits of such a group, and they leave. For others, even the times of fear and grief carry some benefit, and they feel enriched by their contact with other women with breast cancer. Maria W was also keenly aware of the mixture of threat and wisdom this involvement brought.

While hearing these stories makes me realize
how possible it would be for me to be in their place,

they also have brought me to acknowledge the reality that life does go on after a recurrence or mets (metastases) diagnosis. So in the long run, hearing more and more about how women with metastases survive and live their lives makes the whole thing somewhat less scary.

Marjorie volunteers at a local support organization.

> Two volunteers at the Breast Cancer Resource Center where I volunteer have died in the past month. Both were resilient, energetic women who had been doing well, or so I thought. This is a harsh reality check but as long as I remain involved in the world of breast cancer as an activist/volunteer, I'm going to experience this type of loss. I'm still developing coping mechanisms.

Maria B was grateful for her contact with women who have had recurrences, and actually felt this contact had helped her.

> All in all, it has made me less anxious. They are my teachers, my guides, in this living and dying we are all doing all the time. I don't want to die. I don't want pain and enfeeblement, but my fear of dying has a lot of performance anxiety in it. Knowing others, well-loved others, who have developed mets and have died has shown me that if mets comes my way, I, too, will be able to make my way through it and find acceptance and peace, I pray, eventually. There are many fine people in the land of the dead.

Kate felt that she has learned important lessons from the painful experience of others.

> Two friends underwent bone marrow transplant with very harsh side effects. They lost months of

> *what was left of their lives to a therapy that has*
> *since been shown to be no more effective than*
> *standard chemotherapy. That left me angry, very*
> *sad, and much wiser. If I have to face a choice of*
> *risky, experimental treatment, I will know that*
> *bigger is not always better, that the quality of life*
> *is more important than squeezing out every*
> *possible day.*

As for myself, I have learned, over the years, not to personalize the recurrence and disease progression of the women I know and who share their stories with me. I could not do the advocacy work that I do were I to constantly be seeing myself or my future in the lives of the women with metastatic breast cancer I correspond with every day.

As a physician, Ellen learned long ago not to internalize what happens with other patients.

> *If someone I know has a recurrence or dies, it*
> *doesn't increase my anxiety. In a selfish way, I'm*
> *just glad I'm alive. Now that I have an increased*
> *tumor marker, I'm more anxious. I'm concerned*
> *about my partner and about all the living that I*
> *wish still to experience.*

As Sandy, an advocate and fifteen year survivor of Stage III breast cancer, said:

> *I keep it separate from myself. When I have*
> *hotline calls from women with metastatic disease,*
> *I just try to give them what they need…*
> *encouragement, information, a sympathetic ear.*

Learning more about the biology of breast cancer can be helpful in understanding how varied and unique a disease breast cancer really is. On a cellular level, a woman's breast cancer is hers alone, different from that of other breast cancer patients, even though the diagnoses may sound the same. Each woman's cancer has a unique genetic fingerprint, and a unique outcome.

I didn't always understand this, though. When Penny's cancer recurred in the bones of her pelvis seven years after her diagnosis, I was not only devastated for her, but also worried for myself. In our support group, I had always felt a special kinship with Penny. We were temperamentally very much alike. We were both trained as therapists. She was a social worker; I'd been a counselor. We liked to talk about our feelings and experiences, and to help others do so. Within the dynamics of our leaderless support group of nine that tended to drift off into chatting on other subjects, Penny and I often played the role of informal co-facilitators, bringing the focus back to issues that needed to be addressed.

There were other, even more uncanny similarities between us as well. Diagnosed within a month of one another, we had both had large Stage IIA tumors, with no lymph node involvement. We had both had mastectomies and the same chemotherapy protocol, a particularly aggressive version of CMF that had shown superior results in an Italian study. Probably our oncologists had independently read the same journal article a month or two prior to our diagnoses, I later reflected. I've never met anyone before or since who had this same protocol. We also shared an identical sense of betrayal and outrage that our diagnoses had been delayed when our gynecologists had dismissed palpable lumps because they didn't show up on our mammograms. My diagnosis had been delayed for over a year. In Penny's case it was eight months. She took successful legal action, while I decided not to.

The similarities in our disease experience were mere coincidence, I had to remind myself, as I lay awake on the night that she called with the results of her bone scan. There were differences as well. Penny's cancer was lobular, while mine was ductal. And besides, I kept telling myself through my tears, some of us have to survive.

Aches, pains and tears in the night

Symptoms that persist send us all into a state of anxiety. How long should we wait before calling the doctor? Could this be something else, and if so, what? In the next chapter, we'll cover some of the common signs and symptoms of recurrence. This section deals with what it feels like for women to live with their fears, to struggle with the questions that go round and round in our minds as we try to go about our lives, and torment us through sleepless nights. Here are some typical stories.

Marjorie hadn't spent much time thinking about recurrence during her treatment.

> *I didn't understand the obsessive behavior and*
> *anxiety about recurrence when I attended a face-*
> *to-face support group shortly after I was diagnosed.*
> *Now I do! Just a few months after treatment ended,*
> *every headache was possible brain mets, every*
> *backache was bone mets. That mindset has*
> *subsided somewhat but never left completely.*

Five years after her diagnosis, Kate found a suspicious lump on her skin. It took her a while to summon up the courage to call.

> *I felt a very firm lump in the scar along my*
> *lumpectomy. It took me a couple of weeks of*
> *prodding and poking before I called the surgeon.*
> *I didn't want to seem like an over-reactor. It seemed*
> *to take forever to get the mammogram, the*

> surgeon's exam, and finally the biopsy. During that
> time I was convinced that I had a recurrence and
> that the recurrence would be very bad news indeed.
> Symptoms of recurrence are much more
> frightening, I think, than finding the original lump.

Dianne also waited to call her doctor, but for a different reason.

> I had the flu last year (remember the flu, when it
> was just the flu?) and had vertigo so badly I
> couldn't stand up. I was sure it was in my brain.
> I didn't tell anyone my fears, until a friend came to
> take me to the doctor and then I just broke down.
> I also had trouble with a blood pressure medication.
> It was giving me panic attacks, making me dizzy,
> you know, the works, and of course, I was sure it
> was the breast cancer. I don't feel embarrassed
> about telling my doctor my symptoms, just out
> and out afraid. I don't want to hear any more
> bad news.

Emma's oncologist recognized and understood her fear.

> I developed really persistent stabbing pain in the
> incision and my surgeon ordered a unilateral
> mammogram and (I think) sonogram too. I wasn't
> sure whether this was medically mandated or
> whether he simply understood the nerve-
> wrackedness that breast cancer patients experience.
> When I went back for one check-up and told him
> how anxious I'd become, he said, "Even my patients
> who are twenty years out from surgery get nervous."

Debbie's most recent scare occurred right before I interviewed
her. Because it was still fresh in her mind, she was able to
describe it in great detail.

> *Last week, little bumps began to form on my
> chest, cancer-side, between collarbone and
> mastectomy scar. They fit the profile for skin mets
> perfectly, and did not respond to cortisone cream.
> For two days, that's what I thought I had. My
> reaction was similar to what it's been with other
> scares.*

Deciding to keep her fears to herself, Debbie waited to see what would happen.

> *I did not call my oncologist because I did not
> want to jump the gun and seem alarmist. Yes, I'll
> admit it—embarrassed and reluctant describes it.
> Nor did I say anything to anyone else, including my
> husband and breast cancer pals. I felt the need to
> examine this by myself before involving others.
> Plus, there was enough doubt in my mind that it
> seemed reasonable to wait and not alarm others,
> perhaps needlessly.*

Despite these doubts, Debbie found herself rehearsing her response to recurrence in her mind, as she had done before.

> *When I first noticed them, I was obsessed
> (checking appearance/feel of said bumps every
> spare moment) and scared. I played through in my
> mind the scenario of telling my family, most
> particularly my children (very hardest part) that
> "it" was back.*

This mental rehearsal extended all the way through to the end of her life, as Debbie clarified her choices in her mind.

> *I examined, again, my thoughts about treatment
> of advanced disease (how hard would I be willing
> to push it?), and of most importance to me*

personally—how I would obtain enough seconal to have control over the end, should I feel I needed it. I've done this same basic routine with each scare since diagnosis (lump in neck, high CA15-3, thickening above collarbone, assorted lumps noticed, odd backache, yada yada).

As she was working her way through this harrowing mental process, Debbie was also aware of the times she'd been down this road before.

But with time, as I said, the level of each emotion that comes has ratcheted down somewhat, and the duration has shortened. The most-recent skin-mets scare took only a few hours to progress past the terror/obsession stage, into the reflective. Before the time the bumps faded, I felt fairly confident and able to face "it" with resolve. Sad, but confident.

Bringing the process full circle, Debbie concluded:

Lest this sound too composed, when I woke up to find the bumps almost gone, I lost it—cried, shouted, cried some more, and needed a good hike, singing loudly, to release the strong emotions of— what? Relief of course, but also anger, I guess, at having to go through that hard experience, yet again.

Sometimes we can even laugh about our "freak-outs." Sometimes you have to laugh. No other possible response exists.

When my husband and I were vacationing in the beautiful town of Toledo, Spain, one May, a number of years ago, I spent a day doubled over in severe abdominal pain. By the evening, I was in a panic, half-convinced my cancer had metastasized to my liver, which felt distended and tender.

Tom drove me to the local hospital, where with great pointing and groaning I tried to convey my distress to the very courteous young doctor, who spoke no English. Not for the first time, I regretted my useless years of high-school French. Finally, a lab technician was found who could speak a little English. In tears, I told her what I feared. What ensued was a comedy of misunderstandings, as I tried to say that yes, I was afraid I had liver mets, but no I didn't actually have metastatic breast cancer.

Perhaps, it was diplomatically suggested, I was having a gall bladder attack? I was duly dispatched for an ultrasound, and ten minutes later, the young doctor came back in, all smiles. He has obviously rehearsed what he was about to say: "Señora Mayerrr, what you have, it is wind!"

Tom and I looked each other in bewilderment, and then began to laugh. All this drama over an attack of gas!

CHAPTER 5

Everything You Want to Know About Recurrence

SO, HOW WILL I KNOW if the cancer comes back? What symptoms should I be looking for? Are there different kinds of recurrence, with different outcomes? How long will I be at risk of recurrence? Can I ever consider myself cured? What are the long-term statistics on survival, anyway? And what will happen to me if my breast cancer does metastasize?

These are some of the questions on the minds of women who have had breast cancer. They are also issues many women prefer to avoid. Put more precisely, women may want to know the answer to these questions, but they also *don't* want to know, unless it's really necessary. They're afraid that the answers will only add to their worries, and make it even more difficult to live with the uncertainties of breast cancer. They worry about recurrence, but they're reluctant to talk about it, or find out more about it.

Perhaps that's why so little has been written on this subject, while other post-treatment issues, like concerns over body-image, chemo-induced menopause, and sexuality have been explored more fully.

Maybe you are wondering if you should even read further....

The thing is, whether we discuss them or not, these questions are on our minds. Silence surrounding a threatening subject often bears the full weight of our fearful projections. Often, what we imagine may be worse than the reality. Maybe we think: gosh, if they're not telling me anything and avoiding the issue, it must be pretty bad news. Not knowing what symptoms to look out for can lead some of us to worry about every little ache and pain.

This book takes the position that it is better to talk about it, and have accurate information, at least for those of us who tend to magnify fears in the absence of knowledge. And maybe it's not only the anxious information seekers like myself who can benefit from opening this dark door and shining a light inside to see what is there. Maybe it will be helpful to you, too.

This chapter and the next one on follow-up testing contain the information you need to answer all the questions above and more. Both chapters contain stories from women who are living with the same feelings of uncertainty you are facing.

What we don't know

Recurrence is difficult to talk about, and easy to avoid. Perhaps this is why many oncologists are hesitant to volunteer much specific information about recurrence to their patients, and why there are few educational materials out there on this subject. And many patients are afraid to ask. As a consequence, most women who have had breast cancer know very little about recurrence.

"Most patients don't want to know about recurrence," some doctors may say. "Why cause them unnecessary worry?" Doctors who feel this way seem to believe that if they don't mention it, we won't think about it. Perhaps this is true, for many women. But it wasn't for me, and for many women I know.

Dr. Bill Buchholz, a medical oncologist in Mountain View, California, and author of *Live Longer, Live Larger* offers his perspective:

> *When a patient asks for information, I usually ask her how it will be used. I note that some people use it for making decisions, others to allay their fears. If the need is to address fears—and I cannot give useful information—I try to address the fears directly. One concern is overwhelming patients with too much information that does not lead to a solution for their problem.* [1]

Patients are sometimes advised by their doctors to think positively and focus on a good outcome. While well-intentioned and helpful for some women, this kind of advice can fall far short of the mark for others, especially in the early months and years after diagnosis. I have never found being told not to worry particularly helpful—whether that advice comes from a doctor, family member or friend. In fact, it often feels a bit insulting, as if it's being implied that somehow I am choosing negativity and pessimism, when in fact I'm working hard to come to terms with a drastic change in my life.

To those physicians who would have us just cheer up by assuming the best, I would say, trust us to work through our process in our own way. It may take some time, but we will get there. It will help if you are generous with information, when we ask for it.

Observing a reluctance to speak of recurrence in her own caregivers, Emma speculates about why this may be so.

> *I've sensed my doctors are reluctant to talk of such things. They seem to feel my odds of surviving*

> *without recurrence are high enough not to warrant*
> *such talk. But perhaps there is a general reluctance*
> *among doctors to "go there" until it's absolutely*
> *necessary.*

Some women, like Sara W, are comfortable bringing the subject up.

> *I talk openly to my oncologist about recurrence,*
> *and most of my medical records refer to me as "a*
> *slightly anxious woman"! I do consider myself well*
> *informed and don't hesitate to come in for a visit*
> *with a ton of questions.*

However, Adele's experience is more typical of the women I interviewed.

> *When I finished chemo, my oncologist told me*
> *that I should let him know of any difference that*
> *I noticed. He said this in such a way that I*
> *understood that he didn't mean every little ache*
> *and pain but anything really out of the ordinary.*
> *Other than that, we haven't really talked about the*
> *possibility of metastatic disease.*

If they are involved with support groups or organizations, women who've had breast cancer certainly know of women with advanced disease, and may know some who have died. But they may not know much in the way of specifics. Often they imagine the worst: debilitating treatments, and a quick downward spiral toward an imminent death. They aren't aware how treatable metastatic disease often is, or that 21 percent of women who are diagnosed with Stage IV disease survive at least five years.

Remembering a relative who died from cancer in the past, when side effects from chemotherapy and radiation were much more debilitating, women will sometimes indicate that they're not sure they would choose to be treated should they have a recurrence. Why would they want to endure such horrible treatments, they will say, if a cure was no longer possible?

In their minds, a recurrence is a recurrence, since the distinction in prognosis and treatment between a local, a regional and a distant recurrence hasn't been explained to them. They believe that regular scans and tests are crucial once treatment ends, and that the early detection of metastases can possibly save their lives. If those scans aren't done, they often worry they are getting inadequate care geared more toward cost-cutting than saving their lives.

Different kinds of recurrence, different outcomes

The word recurrence can be confusing, because it is used to describe three very different situations, with different outcomes and treatment recommendations.

In general, metastatic sites that are close to the original cancer are termed regional or sometimes locoregional recurrences, while those in other parts of the body are referred to as distant metastases. First, let's discuss local recurrences, which may not be metastases at all.

Local recurrence

Local recurrence can happen when tumor cells from the original cancer left behind by surgery eventually divide and grow to form a detectable tumor. The means of growth is by what is called "direct extension" of the tumor.

A local recurrence in the breast after lumpectomy is not considered metastatic disease. Local recurrence is more common if the woman has not had radiation to the breast following her lumpectomy, or if the tumor has not been completely removed by surgery. This is the reason that good surgical margins are so important. To make sure none of the cancer cells are left behind after the initial surgery, a pathologist examines the tissue surrounding the tumor under a microscope.

A local recurrence is usually treated with "salvage" mastectomy, as doctors often refer to it, although a few women may be able to have a more extensive lumpectomy done. In this case, radiation can generally not be given again, as most women will already have had the maximum recommended dose of radiation after their first lumpectomy.

One extensive study, published in the *Journal of Clinical Oncology,* found that up to 10–20 percent of patients have locally recurrent disease one to nine years after lumpectomy and radiation, although most reports show lower incidence.[2]

The purpose of radiation treatments to the rest of the breast and to the tumor bed is to prevent this kind of local recurrence, but it doesn't always work. So, if your tumor recurs in the same area of your breast where you had your original tumor removed, the chances are good that it is a local recurrence, caused by direct extension of the tumor cells from the original cancer.

It is also possible to develop a new primary breast cancer in the same breast after lumpectomy. Since you've already had breast cancer once, this might be called a recurrence, although biologically, it represents a new and separate event from the original tumor. In this case, the prognosis would have little to do with the original tumor.

Unfortunately, it isn't always possible to tell when a recurrence is truly due to return of the original tumor, or instead to the development of a new cancer. Several of the women I interviewed for this book had local recurrences after lumpectomies, had further surgery, and are currently disease-free, indicating that it is possible to go through this type of recurrence and continue to do very well.

Regional (locoregional) recurrence

Most often, regional recurrences occur in lymph nodes, the chest wall (after the breast has been removed) and surrounding tissue, or skin. Regional recurrences may happen either as a result of direct continuous extension of the tumor, as with local recurrences, or via the lymphatic channels to nearby nodes.

Sites of regional recurrence include the muscles of the chest wall, the remaining axillary nodes under the arm, the internal mammary lymph nodes under the breast bone and between the ribs, those up above the collar bone, known as supraclavicular nodes, and the nodes in the neck. The remaining skin and scar tissue can be affected as well. Inflammatory breast cancer, a rare and fast-growing aggressive form of the disease, usually manifests as areas of reddened skin in a rashlike formation or inflamed-looking area, owing to the invasion of lymphatic system in the skin itself. However, most skin metastases are not of this type.

A regional recurrence is considered more serious than a local recurrence, for it usually indicates that the cancer has spread (metastasized) past the confines of the breast and axillary lymph nodes. It is often, but not always, a harbinger of distant metastases. Aggressive treatment of regional disease can still sometimes bring about a long-term remission that may never end, although it is difficult to know whether this is due to the treatment, or to the indolent (slow-growing) nature of the disease in such cases.

Distant metastases

Distant metastases are considered more serious, and incurable in all but a tiny fraction of cases. When breast cancer cells spread from the primary tumor in the breast through the bloodstream to other parts of the body, establish themselves there, and begin to multiply, they are said to have metastasized distantly.

This raises the possibility that there are probably other, smaller metastatic sites elsewhere that are too small to be detected yet. The most common sites for distant metastases are bone, lungs, liver, soft tissue and brain—although breast cancer can spread to many other sites, throughout the body. When they metastasize, ductal and lobular breast cancer often have different patterns of spread.

Most breast cancer deaths are due to the effects of treatment-resistant distant metastases that grow to interfere with the function of vital organs. This is why treatment for metastatic breast cancer is almost always systemic (body-wide) rather than only localized to the known sites of disease, which are usually indicators of more disease that can't yet be detected.

What kind of symptoms should I be looking for?

Breast cancer patients often develop a heightened awareness of changes in their bodies following the end of treatment. As most of us know, the physiological changes brought about by cancer treatments can be quite dramatic, especially if treatment sends a woman into the abrupt menopause we refer to as "chemopause," when ovarian function is shut down by chemotherapy. In addition to hot flashes and night sweats, aches and pains associated with estrogen loss, possibly exacerbated by hormonal treatment, can make this a confusing and difficult time.

The list of possible menopausal symptoms can be extensive. Women may not know how to discriminate between a worrisome symptom and one that is not serious. While they often realize that their state of mind predisposes them to be more alert about "normal" distress, it's difficult to know which symptoms to take seriously. Edite expressed a common source of confusion among breast cancer patients.

> My greatest question/problem is the possibility
> of recurrence anywhere. And how does one know
> when to be a wimp and go to a physician? Does
> that left side stomach pain indicate something or
> is it just bad food? Does that pain in the back—
> neck—arm—indicate something or is it just a
> muscle strain?

Like Edite, most breast cancer patients aren't sure what kinds of signs and symptoms to be concerned about, and their doctors may not have given them much guidance. Barbie was taken completely by surprise when she had her local recurrence.

> It never occurred to me that I would have cancer
> again after the first time. We did talk about it when
> my local recurrence was diagnosed and at that time
> I learned that a very small percentage of women
> have a recurrence and that I, unfortunately, was
> one of them!

Sara M was encouraged to look for signs of local recurrence by her doctor.

> I was advised to check my incisions and my
> axilla for any unusual lumps or bumps, but no one

> *made any mention ever of what I should look out*
> *for in terms of metastatic disease.*

While some patients do want to know a great deal about recurrence, this can lead to disturbing thoughts and fears. Deborah found herself somewhat grateful her doctor hadn't told her more.

> *I'm a bit of a worrywart and have always*
> *worried about my health. By hearing symptoms*
> *I'm afraid I would start developing those*
> *symptoms, maybe psychosomatically."*

For several women I interviewed who participate in the Breast-Cancer Mailing List, hearing other women discuss symptoms they fear may signal a recurrence can be both reassuring and upsetting. As Francine put it, "I probably know more than is good for me."

Marjorie described the dilemma well.

> *My doctor has walked a fine line between arming*
> *me with information and trying to help me get*
> *on with life. We have discussed (ad nauseam) what*
> *might indicate recurrence. We repeat the discussion*
> *each time since I ask more questions with each*
> *visit.*

In their patient guide, *Follow-Up Care for Breast Cancer,* the American Society of Clinical Oncology list the following signs and symptoms for patients to be aware of.

> *Most recurrent breast cancer is suspected or*
> *found by women themselves, and the majority of*
> *recurrences are detected between scheduled medical*
> *visits. So, once your treatment has ended, it is*
> *important to get appropriate follow-up care.*

- *Chronic bone pain or tenderness*

- *Skin rashes, redness, or swelling*

- *New lumps or other changes in your breasts or on your chest*

- *Chest pain, shortness of breath*

- *Persistent abdominal pain*

- *Changes in weight, especially weight loss*[3]

But what is the definition of chronic? What does persistent mean? Hours? Days? Weeks? Dr. Susan Love offers this commonsense advice:

> *If you have pain that lasts for more than a week or two and doesn't seem to be going away, and isn't like whatever pains have been familiar to you in your life, you should get it checked out.*[4]

Any pain unexplained by some other injury or cause that persists for more than two weeks should be investigated, says oncologist Bill Buchholz, adding the caveat that, "a severe pain or symptom should be checked out promptly because it is severe." As a guide to help determine when to call the doctor, Dr. Buchholz advises his patients:

> *Ask yourself the following questions: What would a prudent person do who did not have cancer? What would I do if I were not fearful of cancer? What would I do if I were not fearful of being judged or criticized?*[5]

The National Cancer Institute's PDQ advises the following:

> *A woman who has had cancer in one breast should report any changes in the treated area or in the other breast to her doctor right away. Because a*

> woman who has had breast cancer is at risk of
> getting cancer in the other breast, mammograms
> are an important part of follow-up care.
>
> Also, a woman who has had breast cancer should
> tell her doctor about other physical problems, such
> as pain, loss of appetite or weight, changes in
> menstrual cycles, unusual vaginal bleeding, or
> blurred vision. She should also report headaches,
> dizziness, shortness of breath, coughing or
> hoarseness, backaches, or digestive problems that
> seem unusual or that don't go away. These
> symptoms may be a sign that the cancer has
> returned, but they can also be signs of various other
> problems. It's important to share these concerns
> with a doctor.

The ASCO Guidelines and the NCI statement refer to the most common scenarios for metastatic recurrence, but they do not, of course, constitute a complete list of all possible symptoms that might be indicative of a problem. No such list could be drawn up, nor would it be useful to you. As Dr. Bill Buchholz quite reasonably points out:

> It is literally impossible to prepare for all
> outcomes, or even describe them. Doctors don't
> always understand what is being asked. There is a
> responsibility of the patient, too, to be clear in
> communication and ask for what she wants.

So if something seems out of the ordinary to you, call your oncologist for an appointment to check it out. That's what your doctors are there for, and they expect you to report symptoms that occur between office visits—this is how most metastases are detected. Don't feel you must wait until your next regular appointment, which may be months away. When you talk with your doctor, be as specific as you can by reporting when the symptom occurs, how it feels, and what makes it better or worse.

If you are no longer seeing an oncologist, make sure the doctor you do see knows you have had breast cancer, and doesn't easily dismiss the possibility of recurrence. There are too many stories where pain or other symptoms are never thoroughly evaluated, often because the patient is some years past diagnosis, and the possibility of recurrence isn't considered—not by patient or doctor. Your concern about ruling out recurrence should be addressed in a timely way, and taken seriously. It's important to realize that most recurrences are found by the patient herself presenting with symptoms between scheduled follow-up appointments.

In fact, in a 1991 review of five studies on the effect of routine follow-up on the course of recurrent breast cancer, it was found that symptoms developed between visits in 75 percent to 95 percent of the patients who actually had recurrences. Physicians detected abnormalities in only 15 percent of these recurrent patients with no symptoms.

It's important to note that we are also subject to all the other health concerns that aging women face, and it can sometimes be difficult for us and our physicians to sort out these symptoms from those of metastatic breast cancer.

Some women may be concerned about "bothering" their oncologists with symptoms, and don't want to be seen as complainers. Consequently, when a symptom presents itself, there's not only the worry about the symptom, but also a concern about how they will be perceived. Edite expressed a common feeling.

> When I visit the oncologist I really never know
> how to answer his, "How are you?" Do I complain

about that niggling cough, nagging pain or will he
think I am becoming a hypochondriac? It would
be nice to have a list: with this symptom see a
physician if it continues for four weeks or more;
with this symptom see a physician if it continues for
more than two days; with this symptom see a
physician immediately. Then there would be some
peace of mind.

How long will I be at risk of recurrence?

Some other kinds of cancer grow so rapidly and aggressively that if the initial treatments don't work and the disease recurs, it almost always comes back very soon, within a year or two. So few patients survive initially that recurrences are unusual. Consequently, if a patient who has one of these cancers is still disease-free after a few years, he or she is usually considered cured.

Breast cancer tends not to behave in this way. As we've seen, recurrence can still happen over two decades, and even more, in rare cases. However, when breast cancer does recur, it often does so in the early years after diagnosis. According to the ASCO *Patient Guide* cited above, between 60 percent and 80 percent of all breast cancer recurrences are detected within three years after treatment ends.

Looking at patterns of recurrence, researchers Michael Baum, of the University College in London, and Romano Demicheli, of the Instituto Tumori in Milan, independently arrived at the same "bimodal" or double peaked curve, indicating when first metastases occur after diagnosis. The first peak for early metastases happened at 18–24 months after diagnosis, followed by a broader late metastases peak at five years, which gradually decreased over many years.[6]

This is why, when it comes to breast cancer, there are no absolute guarantees of cure after treatment. It simply isn't possible to reduce risk of recurrence to zero—to say positively that you are cured as of this moment and there is no chance you will ever have to worry about breast cancer again. There is no magical five-year or ten-year point in time when breast cancer can be described as cured. For women who are living with N.E.D. (no evidence of disease) there is only a steadily declining risk.

The concept of risk is often misunderstood. People tend to think about risk as if it were a standard light switch—it's either on or it's off. You are either at risk or you're not at risk. But risk is actually more like a dimmer switch, with an infinite series of probabilities between high, low and no risk.

The fact of the matter is, when we make treatment choices, we have to settle for risk *reduction,* not risk elimination. It's the same thing with looking at risk for recurrence, an imponderable figure that can never be known for sure, but that's always changing depending upon your prognosis and your time since diagnosis.

The only way we can find out when recurrences happen with modern treatments is from clinical trials in which different treatment regimens have been compared, and then women are followed over a period of time—usually five or ten years. When we look at data like this, however, it's important not to compare apples and oranges. The women in the study must have had the same kind and stage of disease, and the same treatments as you have had, for the figures to be meaningful for you. And even when these conditions apply, it's important to know that there's a range of outcomes for any group of women with similar stage and treatment choices. No one can tell you where you, personally, might fall within that range.

Because they can vary so widely depending upon prognosis, these estimates are best tailored to each individual woman. The prognosis (and the staging done at initial diagnosis) will be based on the size and other pathology of the tumor, the extensiveness of lymph node involvement, if any, and the presence of regional or distant metastases. This is the TNM (tumor, node, metastasis) model that your oncologist or surgeon used to assign a stage to your cancer. In addition, the pathology of your tumor will have been assessed, which includes hormone receptor status, HER2 expression or amplification, measures of tumor grade and proliferative rate, and other factors.

A complete explanation of the staging system is available at the National Cancer Institute website *http://www.cancer.gov/cancer_information/cancer_type/breast/* or by calling (800) 422-6237.

Don't look back

When you were diagnosed, your oncologist gave you the best information available at that time about recurrence rates for your stage and kind of breast cancer, with or without various treatment options. Usually the figures available show disease-free survival over five or ten years. In this way, you were able to estimate how the various treatment options were likely to improve the odds that you would survive without distant metastatic recurrence, for at least that period of time. This in turn helped you to decide whether the potential side effects of the treatments you were offered were outweighed by the likely benefits.

Not every woman will choose to have such a detailed, in-depth conversation with her oncologist, of course, but knowing your personal risks and benefits from treatment can ensure that you are a full partner in the decision-making process, and that you made the best treatment decisions for you at the time.

It's not uncommon for subsequent research to alter treatment recommendations a year or two or five after your treatment. When newer research findings are trumpeted in the media, patients treated at an earlier point in time may worry that they may not have received the best treatment.

I've had to confront this several times over the years since my diagnosis—and this is likely to happen to any primary breast cancer patient who decides to stay current on the research in adjuvant treatment for breast cancer.

Not long after my chemotherapy was completed, a large, well-designed clinical trial showed that even for patients who had hormone receptor negative breast cancers like mine, taking tamoxifen could reduce the risk of a contralateral breast cancer—a new cancer in the other breast—by as much as 50 percent. Since I'd had a hysterectomy years earlier, I wasn't at risk for endometrial cancer, and as far as I knew ran no increased risk for stroke or other clotting disorder. On the strength of that finding, because I knew I was at increased risk for another cancer, my oncologist and I decided that I should take tamoxifen, which I tolerated reasonably well, with no serious side effects.

Not long after my five years of tamoxifen was up, another new study established that there was no benefit after all for tamoxifen for ER-negative breast cancer patients and perhaps even a small detriment in rates of recurrence. The study recommended against its use. It's not uncommon for studies of the same research question to arrive at different findings, which is why multiple studies are usually needed. Of course, I wasn't happy that I had exposed myself to the risks and side effects of tamoxifen for five years, for little if any hope of benefit. But I took some comfort in the fact that I had made the best decision I could, with the knowledge available to me, at the time.

My experience is far from unique. Many patients end up having to cope with some degree of regret about their treatment choices, either because they've learned information subsequently that might have informed earlier decisions, or because the treatments themselves have changed. Issues of delayed diagnosis and medical malpractice aside, I have found that reaffirming, "I made the best decision I could at the time" becomes a crucial coping tool. As much as possible, I think it's important to avoid second-guessing your treatment decisions, whatever the outcome. Coping with breast cancer is tough enough without also having to shoulder the bitterness and regret that persistent feelings of "if only" can invite into your life.

Science marches forward, inevitably, taking some false turnings in the process. There are continuous incremental refinements in treatment being made—and sometimes a brand new treatment or treatment combination will lead to a major change. Yet we usually don't have the luxury of waiting for medical certainty when we make our treatment decisions. We must act when we must act, with the most current information available at that point in time. And that information, like everything else around us, is constantly changing.

Long-term statistics on survival

We know that breast cancer can be a slow-growing disease, and that even when it metastasizes, some patients can live for many years, with good quality of life. We also know that while the prognoses for different stages and kinds of breast cancer are very different, generally the only long-term figures (more than ten years) that we have are aggregate, meaning all breast cancer cases are lumped together. This makes it very hard to come up with good individual estimates of survival.

The importance of understanding the variability in outcomes for each individual patient was eloquently expressed by the late evolutionary biologist and author, Stephen Jay Gould, in his essay, *The Median is Not the Message,*[7] a classic exploration of statistics that ought to be required reading for every cancer patient.

When Gould was diagnosed in 1982 with a rare and deadly abdominal cancer known as mesothelioma, his doctor told him that there was "nothing really worth reading" in the medical literature. Undeterred, he did a library computer search on his disease. "I realized with a gulp why my doctor had offered that humane advice," Gould wrote. "The literature couldn't have been more brutally clear: mesothelioma is incurable, with a median mortality of only eight months after discovery."

Most people, unschooled in statistics, would think that this meant that they had only eight months to live. As a scientist, Gould knew better. The median describes that point in a distribution that separates the cases in half. Half the people lived fewer than eight months, and half lived for a longer time.

Like the mean (average) or mode (most common score), the median is only an abstraction—what is called a "measure of central tendency." Yet we tend to see such a measure as the one essential truth to be extracted from that statistic. "We still carry the historical baggage of a Platonic heritage that seeks sharp essences and definite boundaries," Gould explained, adding that we tend to see the mean and median as "the hard realities, and the variation that permits their calculation as a set of transient and imperfect measurements of this hidden essence." In fact, the opposite is true. "All evolutionary biologists know that variation itself is nature's only irreducible essence. Variation is the hard reality."

Now that he knew that half the people with his disease would live longer than eight months, Gould set about determining the shape of the distributional curve, and in fact found it was what statisticians call "right skewed," meaning that some patients lived on for many years. Why not he?

Just as important, the statistics had been based on conventional treatment. With a new experimental protocol and the best medical care, he might well outlive even the best predictions. "I had obtained," Gould concluded, "in all probability, the most precious of all possible gifts in the circumstances—substantial time." Gould died twenty years later, of an unrelated cancer.

Then and now

The best overall statistics on long-term cancer survival we have in the United States, as we've indicated earlier in discussing the concept of "cure," come from the Surveillance, Epidemiology, and End Results (SEER) Program of the National Cancer Institute (NCI), tracking survival and mortality over the last quarter century. While these figures may be limited in scope, I'm including them here because so many women with breast cancer either over- or underestimate what true long-term survival from the disease really is.

If women read only what I (perhaps over-critically) refer to as the "pink ribbon propaganda," they may conclude that the 97 percent five-year survival of breast cancer "caught early" means that all but a very few women ultimately survive the disease. If they hang out in support groups, online and elsewhere, where there's a preponderance of women with high-risk and active metastatic disease, and hear people say repeatedly that breast cancer can never be cured, they may conclude that all but a very few breast cancer patients die of the disease in the end.

I've heard both perceptions expressed many times. Neither one tells the real story. Based on the most recent SEER data, relative survival rates (adjusted for other causes of death) for women diagnosed with invasive breast cancer are: 86 percent at 5 years, 76 percent after 10 years, 58 percent after 15 years, 53 percent after 20 years, and 50 percent after 25 years.[8]

These figures can be described as both relevant and outdated. Obviously, we can't know, for sure, what the 25-year survival of a woman diagnosed today with breast cancer will be, so most statisticians will go back into the past to see how women did who were diagnosed 20 or 25 years ago. The problem is that so much has changed in the world of breast cancer since that time.

A woman diagnosed with breast cancer over a quarter century ago, in 1975, faced very different treatments than she does today. A different disease paradigm still prevailed then, although it was about to change. In that era, it was widely believed that cancer traveled from the breast through the regional nodes and surrounding tissue in a predictable, orderly fashion when it metastasized, so the more tissue you removed, the greater the likelihood of cure.

Consequently, a woman diagnosed as late as the early 1970's was likely to have a disfiguring radical mastectomy, removing not only her breast and axillary nodes, but also the muscles of her chest wall. She was far less likely to receive any chemotherapy, radiation or hormonal treatment, unless her cancer was locally advanced or metastatic. Tamoxifen was a new drug and relatively untested then. Only in the last few years has it been known that tamoxifen is effective in premenopausal women as well as in postmenopausal women. The notion that additional systemic treatment after surgery (adjuvant therapy) can prevent or delay many recurrences is a relatively recent concept, at least on a time scale of decades.

Today, in the United States, the standard recommendation for most invasive breast cancers of at least 1 centimeter (and sometimes smaller, if there is unfavorable pathology) will be for adjuvant hormonal treatment and/or combination chemotherapy if the patient is premenopausal or her tumor is hormone receptor negative. In some parts of Europe, and elsewhere among developed nations, adjuvant chemotherapy is still used more sparingly.

In multiple randomized clinical trials, adjuvant treatments have been shown to moderately decrease recurrence and save lives, confirming the paradigm that breast cancer can spread through the bloodstream as well as the lymphatic system, and that it is often systemic even when a tumor is small and apparently localized. Long-term survival data has confirmed that lumpectomy with radiation is equivalent to mastectomy.

The nature of breast cancer diagnosed in American women has steadily been changing over the years. The most dramatic change, of course, is that women are being diagnosed at earlier and earlier stages of the disease, largely because of campaigns for early detection, mammography screening, breast self-examination and awareness. This is having some impact on mortality, although not nearly as much as had been hoped, as we'll see later in this chapter.

The trend toward earlier detection is much more pronounced in Caucasian women, while African-American women are still diagnosed at later stages, and die in disproportionally greater numbers, even though their breast cancer incidence is lower.

In the past decade, the stigma about breast cancer has lifted, so that women are much less likely to conceal the disease or feel shame about having it. Consequently, these changes in treatment and in stage at diagnosis make extrapolating survival and mortality information from the past into the present somewhat problematic. Nevertheless, it is the data we have, and worth looking at with these caveats in mind.

Conditional survival and period analysis

Traditionally, estimates of prognosis and survival are made at the time of diagnosis, but this may not be the only way to look at survival, nor even the most accurate way. Survival estimates, it turns out, are dynamic, and actually change over time. One way to express this is known as "conditional survival."

Conditional survival takes into account the median length of time since diagnosis, and generally finds that the longer the time a patient has already survived after an initial critical period, the longer she is likely to survive. This is true because most of those likely to die of the disease have recurrences and die in the early years after diagnosis—the initial critical period. Conditional survival is particularly meaningful with advanced and high-risk cancers, which tend to recur sooner. The study authors of a 2001 analysis of conditional median survival in metastatic cancers found that, "as cancer patients survive, their survival estimate is constantly changing."[9]

As we'll see demonstrated graphically later in this chapter, the risk for recurrence isn't spread evenly out over time. Most metastatic recurrences will happen in the early years after diagnosis. While no one can provide you with a specific prediction for how long you as an individual will live, or how likely you are to have a recurrence, it has been very helpful to me to realize that the longer I live with no recurrence, the better my chances of continuing to live on disease-free are likely to be.

Recently, a mathematical technique known as "period analysis," used in actuarial projections, has been proposed as a way of correcting survival figures that that they reflect improvements in treatment and early detection over time.

The work of German statistician Hermann Brenner with period analysis, offers us what may turn out to be a more accurate—and certainly more positive—way to look at survival statistics taken from the US SEER data.[10] This method takes into account the interim survival data for patients diagnosed in later years as a correction for the original survival data of a particular "cohort" of women diagnosed twenty years ago. Using this technique, Dr. Brenner has found that the twenty year period relative survival for invasive breast cancer is 65 percent, an improvement from the "cohort" relative survival figure of 52 percent. Figure 5-1 presents this data in graphic terms.

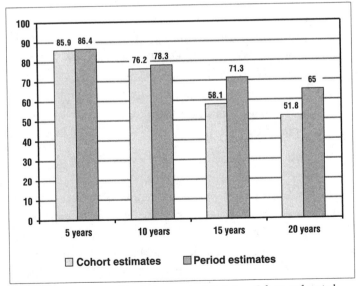

Figure 5-1. 20 years SEER relative survival statistics: Cohort and period analysis (Data from H Brenner, Lancet, October 2002, analysis)

If these figures hold up, they suggest that an average patient diagnosed and treated today with invasive breast cancer is substantially more likely to survive fifteen or twenty years after diagnosis than would a patient who was diagnosed two decades ago.

When do first recurrences happen?

One way to look at risk for and timing of recurrence is to look at the outcomes of large groups of breast cancer patients over extended periods of time. A 1999 study of all patients with invasive breast cancer listed in the University of Chicago tumor registry looked at recurrences in 1,547 patients treated with mastectomies between 1945 and 1987, a span of over forty years. The study found that:

> *Most recurrences occurred within the first ten years after mastectomy. Recurrences were rare after twenty years; only one recurrence was reported among 192 patients followed for 26–45 years. Patients who had a recurrence within five years following mastectomy had shorter subsequent survival times than those whose recurrence appeared after five years.*[11]

The problem with these figures, as we've indicated already, is that treatment has changed dramatically since 1987, and even more so during the twenty years before that. Since most women with invasive breast cancer now receive adjuvant chemotherapy, hormonal treatment, or both, not only has this improved long-term survival, but it also may have extended the length of remission in women who do end up having metastatic recurrences.

Nevertheless, Figure 5-2 gives an immediate sense of the shape of the curve of first recurrence incidence over time. The figures include both regional and distant recurrences, but exclude local recurrences. It's clear that in this study, the overwhelming number of first recurrences happened in the early years after diagnosis, reinforcing the concept of conditional survival.

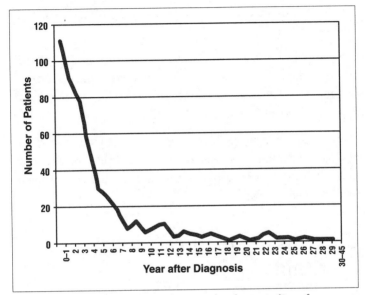

Figure 5-2. When first recurrences happen after diagnosis (Data from University of Chicago "Dormancy" study of 1,547 breast cancer patients diagnosed 1945–87, excludes local recurrences)

Because an estimated 97 percent of metastatic breast cancer patients will ultimately die of their disease, mortality rates indirectly reflect rates of distant recurrence. Due to length of survival with recurrence, however, mortality occurs later. The SEER mortality data paints a similar picture, going back a quarter century. It tells us that for breast cancer patients diagnosed in 1975 who developed metastatic disease and died in the intervening years, the largest percentage (31 percent) died within the first five years after diagnosis.

About an equal number (29 percent) died in each of the next five-year periods—five to ten years and ten to fifteen years after diagnosis. A much smaller—but still significant—percentage (11 percent) died between fifteen and twenty years after diagnosis. It can be said that either they had late recurrences, or that they lived with metastatic breast cancer for significant periods of time—or both.

Overall, the mortality rate (expressed in the SEER data per 100,000 population) from breast cancer has fallen about 13 percent since 1982, and continues to decrease in recent years at a rate in excess of 3 percent each year.

Even though we can't really tell from survival figures how much of this improvement is related to earlier detection, and how much to better treatment or other factors in the lives of women, this is still good news.

Changes in breast cancer over time

How has breast cancer changed over time, both in terms of stage at diagnosis and deaths?

Figure 5-3 is based on a 2002 *New York Times* article interviewing Dr. Barnett Kramer, director of the Office of Disease Prevention at the National Institutes of Health. It offers us a snapshot of the increases in incidence of earlier stages of breast cancer in recent years, coupled with the much more modest decreases in later stage disease. The figures represent rates of incidence per 100,000 people, and are corrected for age and size of the population. Science journalist Gina Kolata puts the matter succinctly.

> *If screening worked perfectly, every cancer found early would correspond to one fewer cancer found*

	Rate per 100,000 population		Change over 15 year period
	1983	1998	Rate & percent change per 100,000 population
DCIS	6	31	+25 ↑ 503%
Small localized tumors	22	60	+38 ↑ 273%
Large localized tumors (> 2 cm.)	27	24	−3 ↓ 11%
Lymph node positive tumors	42	38	−4 ↓ 9%
Stage IV (distant metastases)	4.3	3.7	No trend (P = 0.83)
Deaths from breast cancer	32	28	−4 ↓ 13%

Figure 5-3. Changes in stage at diagnosis and deaths from breast cancer (SEER Data United States, 1983–1998)

> *later. That, he [Kramer] said, did not happen.*
> *Mammography instead has resulted in a huge new*
> *population of women with early stage cancer but*
> *without a corresponding decline in the numbers of*
> *women with advanced cancer.[12]*

The good news here is that large, localized tumors and lymph node positive tumors—both at higher risk of recurring—are somewhat less common than they were years ago, at least among white women. While these modest decreases in high-risk diagnoses are evident, the incidence of breast cancer overall has continued to rise, disproportionately, as indicated by the large increases in early stage breast cancers and DCIS.

Clearly, not all of these early cancers, if left undetected until a later time, would have progressed to become fatal. Many more of the cancers being found now through mammography will turn out to lack the capacity to become metastatic, or even invasive, but we don't yet have a way to assess this—yet.

My own hope is that we will see the end of "one-size-fits-all" and "just-in-case" treatments in breast cancer, and that new kinds of tests will give us the ability to discriminate so well between different types of breast cancer that patients will no longer have to receive treatments which they don't need and from which they are unlikely to benefit. Scientists are hopeful that within a few years, gene expression profiling and proteomics, through the use of microarrays and other analytic tools, will lead to the first truly accurate prognostic (outcome) and predictive (treatment response) assessment we've had in breast cancer. But for right now, treatment is still offered to everyone, because we're still not sure how to tell the difference between those who are at serious risk of recurrence and those who are not.

Many women decide early on in their recovery process that statistics based on group outcomes don't serve them very well or represent their individual situations. They may have found themselves tormented by the numbers their oncologists have reluctantly given to them—and in rejecting an obsessive concern with these figures, they've dismissed the whole notion of predictive statistics altogether.

It's been my experience that a thoughtful statistical perspective can be of real help to women who are coping with a breast cancer diagnosis, and wondering—as we inevitably do—about prognosis. I hope you will be able to take away from this discussion a few numbers and concepts that address your own concerns.

CHAPTER 6

Follow-up Testing: Fears, Facts and Fallacies

IT'S IMPORTANT to find a recurrence as early as possible—isn't it? So, why isn't my doctor doing routine scans and tumor markers?

Women are confused about how much and what kind of routine testing should be a part of their medical care after a breast cancer diagnosis. If they're not having tumor markers and scans, they may worry that cost-saving measures are interfering with their best chance for early detection of metastatic disease. Why should they still be getting mammograms, but not have these other tests done? And if they are getting tested, they may have misconceptions about what the tests are capable of showing.

This chapter focuses on questions related to follow-up testing after breast cancer treatment, an area that is fraught with misunderstanding. More specifically, the focus is on routine follow-up testing for the purpose of detecting metastases in women who have no symptoms of recurrence.

First, patients themselves share their attitudes, fears and experiences about the follow-up tests they undergo. Next, we review the kinds of tests currently available for this purpose, and how well they work, as well as newer tests that are becoming more widely available. The randomized clinical trials that have examined the issue of follow-up testing are explored, as well as the patient guidelines from the American Society for Clinical Oncology and the Canadian Medical Association. Since clinical exams and patient histories represent the best method for finding a recurrence, the guidelines for what constitutes a good clinical exam are discussed. Finally, we explore the emotional costs of maintaining a state of vigilance.

Testing and the search for reassurance

Most breast cancer patients who have finished their treatment assume they will be tested to make sure their cancer has not recurred. When this testing doesn't occur, they may be dismayed and worried, as Deborah was.

> *After I finished chemo I questioned why my oncologist didn't do all the bone scans and blood tests that I've heard about. The answers surprised me. I've been told that symptoms of mets show up just as quickly as finding mets with the tests. I've been told that the survival rate is the same if you do the tests or don't do them. Intuitively I can't get there in my mind. I feel that by using the tests to find out I would get to it earlier, thus slow things down earlier.*

Deborah shares this confusion with many thousands of other breast cancer patients who are looking to testing for periodic reassurance that their cancer hasn't recurred. If they're going to go through the anxiety of frequent clinical exams, they reason, why can't they have the tests that will rule out recurrence? At least then, they would know they were okay at that point in time.

Kate, too, was struggling with the absence of follow-up testing.

> *I have a mammogram annually now. Nothing*
> *else is done, although I wish I did have a chest*
> *x-ray and bone scan more often. I've had both*
> *when symptoms were present—a persistent cough*
> *and shortness of breath and back pain. Although*
> *I know that the back pain is degenerative arthritis*
> *and the shortness of breath the beginnings of*
> *chronic pulmonary disease, it is hard not to think*
> *"cancer." At the same time, I don't want a lot*
> *of useless tests that would only take time, energy,*
> *and resources and not mean anything.*

Marjorie's doctor had ordered a number of scans for her.

> *I just had my annual bone and CT scan. I think*
> *my oncologist wants to watch me closely based on*
> *the pathology of the cancer. My latest follow up*
> *scan has shown "something" in my lungs. I just had*
> *a fairly bad head cold and maybe it was related to*
> *that. I'm not planning my funeral but I haven't*
> *slept well since learning about this and won't feel*
> *at ease until I have a PET scan to prove I'm okay.*

Why do Deborah and Kate have no routine tests to detect recurrence, while Marjorie does? Are they correct in their view of testing as a source of potential reassurance? Isn't it important to find a recurrence as early as possible?

Tests beget tests

It seems like such a simple, intuitively appealing idea, undergoing tests to rule out recurrence. Studies have shown that most patients, when asked, would prefer to be tested. And why not?

One reason why not is that if there are findings of any kind, one thing can quickly lead to another, and women can find themselves caught up in a whole series of anxiety-provoking tests, over extended periods of time. This is a common experience.

When my oncologist stopped ordering an annual chest x-ray a few years ago, I remembered having read in the paper that chest x-rays didn't do a very good job at early detection of lung cancer. By the time they found a lung cancer on an x-ray, in most cases it had already spread—so there turned out to be no survival benefit. All these years, I'd assumed I was getting the chest x-ray to rule out lung metastases.

Still, I felt safe. I was still getting my tumor markers tested twice a year, although I'd long ago weaned myself from the anxious habit of calling a week or two after my six-month visits, just to be sure the numbers were within the normal range. I knew my oncologist was monitoring me with these tests, and therefore I could trust that I was cancer-free.

It turns out that isn't quite the case. Whatever patients perceive or wish these tests to show, the realities are quite different. Dr. Charles Loprinzi, of the Mayo Clinic, has written and researched follow-up testing in breast cancer, and understands the pitfalls well.

> *Clinicians well know that "normal" test results are the results seen in "most" healthy people, but there are many healthy people who have test findings that are outside of the normal range. Along this line, the more*

> *tests that are obtained in a normal, healthy person, the more likely it is that one or more of the tests will fall outside of the normal range.*[1]

My own love-hate relationship with testing came to a head about two years ago, when my oncologist referred me to a cardiologist because of some minor chest pain I had while exercising. A stress test showed nothing, nor did a thallium stress test, where a radioactive isotope helped with imaging the blood vessels.

The next step in conventional testing would have been an angiogram, but that carried some risk, and seemed unnecessarily invasive to both the doctor and me.

"It's probably indigestion," said the cardiologist, unconcernedly. But if I wanted a further level of certainty, he told me, there was a new test available, called an ultra-fast CT scan of the heart. It would not be covered by insurance, but it would show any calcium deposits in the arteries around my heart. Calcium was often, but not always, a component of arterial plaque, he explained. The test wasn't infallible, hadn't been shown to save lives or reduce heart attack risk, but it was quick, relatively inexpensive, and non-invasive. I went ahead with the scan, without a thought in the world about how it might relate to my breast cancer history.

My coronary arteries were, blessedly, completely clear of calcium deposits. But in the report, the radiologist made notations about nodules in my lungs. And there were unexplained "densities" in my liver, all within the visual field of the CT scan. I remember sitting there with the report in my hand, my heart pounding. I could feel the blood draining from my face. Now what? I had no symptoms, and felt fine. Or I had until I'd read the test results.

My oncologist thought the lung nodules would likely be from my smoking history, although I'd quit 25 years before. He recommended an MRI of my liver, to further investigate the "densities." Two weeks later, lying on my back, waiting for the tech to slide me into the narrow MRI tube, I remember looking up through the skylight at the leaves of the trees above, moving in the wind, and tried to banish the dark thoughts from my mind.

More days later came the definitive answer: I had hepatic cysts, a benign condition that probably would never cause me any problems. Mixed in with the huge sense of relief was a growing conviction that this sequence of tests, and the weeks of anxiety attending them, had probably been unnecessary. Yet once set in motion, the progression of events had been impossible to stop.

One lesson this experience has taught me is that the more one looks, the more one is likely to find, and the more further testing will be done, often at great cost—not only in resources and dollars, but in emotional distress.

At a 2002 meeting of the Radiological Society of North America, Dr. Giovanna Casola, of the University of California at San Diego, presented the results of a study of 1,192 patients ages 22 to 85 who had full-body scans at private, for-profit imaging centers, many of which aggressively market their services to the worried well, despite the fact that the benefit of these scans in otherwise healthy patients is unproven. Forty-six per cent of the scans in this study showed abnormalities, most in the lungs, kidneys or liver, and 36 percent of patients were advised to have follow-up testing. According to Casola, previous research has shown that scan-detected abnormalities are usually insignificant.[2]

How useful were all these follow-up tests for breast cancer patients, anyway, I wondered? How much did they actually tell us? Did they actually save lives by starting treatment sooner? I began reading the research with a newfound interest.

I am part of several breast cancer networks, and so I started to ask other women I knew about their routine follow-up care post-treatment. I discovered that oncologists vary widely in their testing recommendations. Some employed aggressive monitoring, including a full battery of tests, especially for their Stage II or III patients. I learned that follow-up testing was more likely to be done the first several years after treatment, the period when recurrences are most likely. This battery of tests typically included a complete blood count and blood chemistry, tumor markers (CA 15-3, CA 27.29 and/or CEA), bone scans, liver ultrasound, chest x-ray and computerized tomography (CT) or magnetic resonance imagery (MRI) of the chest, abdomen and pelvis. More recently, there had been some use of PET (positron emission tomography) scans.

But many more doctors, I learned, were no longer ordering these tests for their breast cancer patients who were doing well, without symptoms, after treatment had ended. These oncologists relied exclusively on periodic clinical examinations and histories, in addition to the patients' own reports either between visits or during examinations, for detection of metastatic breast cancer. When asked about this strategy, they reassured their patients that most recurrences were found this way, and not through routine testing.

I couldn't help wondering if this practice was really safe. How could a woman be sure this refusal to test wasn't yet another example of the reduction of services championed by managed care? Or was there something I was missing, something about the tests themselves, or the disease? Clearly, I needed to dig a little deeper.

According to research published in 1994, about 85 percent of recurrent metastatic disease is detected by history and physical exams by the oncologist, or by the patient's own reports to the doctor of symptoms.[3] As Dr. Clifford Hudis, Chief of the Breast Cancer Medical Service at Memorial Sloan-Kettering Cancer Center in New York City puts it, "This suggests that the most important thing you can do is to talk to patients every three to four months and find out if anything is bothering them."[4]

All well and good, I thought. But I still couldn't see what was wrong with adding on some tests to pick up that 15 percent. Wouldn't they offer an additional degree of confidence? And simply asking patients how they felt seemed so low-tech and unscientific, somehow. So I began reading about the tests themselves, and what they were used for.

In any discussion of medical testing, you're likely to encounter the terms *sensitivity* and *specificity*. In the kinds of tests we're discussing here, a test that is highly *sensitive* will do a good job of finding metastases if they are there, and yield very few false negatives—that's when you're told the test is negative, but it really isn't. A highly sensitive test will be good at ruling out disease. When a test is described as highly *specific* for metastatic disease, that means it does a good job of finding patients who are free of disease, and yields very few false-positives—that's when you're told the test is positive when it really isn't. A test with high specificity will not have multiple causes for positive findings. So, when a test has both high sensitivity and specificity, if a woman tests positive it means she has metastases, and when she tests negative, it means she is disease free.

Chest x-rays

A chest x-ray can potentially show metastases in the lung or in the bone, where they appear as dark areas. However, chest x-rays have a rather dismal track record at actually finding cancerous lesions in asymptomatic patients.

A 1989 Danish study that followed 263 primary breast cancer patients with nearly 1,600 x-rays over seven years, found only four metastases in patients with no symptoms. In other words, only one quarter of 1 percent of the chest x-rays found a metastasis that had no symptoms, and there were an equal number of false positives.[5]

A 1983 Italian study of 1,700 patients who received 11,000 chest x-rays over nine years, found even fewer asymptomatic metastases, only a tiny fraction of one percent, but noted "A small gain of three months, not statistically significant, of mean life from metastases diagnosis was recorded for asymptomatic cases, which is probably entirely due to the lead time effect of anticipated diagnosis." In other words, these patients didn't actually live any longer. They just knew they had metastatic disease for three months longer.[6]

As an avid information-seeker who prides herself on facing hard realities, my knee-jerk response had always been that of course I would want to be among those who got the bad news at the earliest possible moment. Reading this, I wasn't so sure.

Tumor markers

Tumor markers are factors in the blood produced by the cancer itself or by the body responding to the tumor. According to a Fact Sheet from the National Cancer Institute,

> *Measurements of tumor marker levels alone are not sufficient to diagnose cancer for the following reasons:*
>
> - *Tumor marker levels can be elevated in people with benign conditions.*
>
> - *Tumor marker levels are not elevated in every person with cancer—especially in the early stages of the disease.*
>
> - *Many tumor markers are not specific to a particular type of cancer; the level of a tumor marker can be raised by more than one type of cancer.*[7]

The tumor markers CA 15-3, CA 27.29, CA 125 and CEA have been widely used to monitor metastatic cancers, especially as a useful early indicator in assessing whether a treatment is successful or not when women are in active therapy for their advanced breast cancer. Tumor markers are not elevated in all metastatic cancer patients, however. One German study found CA 15-3 elevated in 73 percent of women with metastatic breast cancer.[8]

CEA has been shown to be more useful in colorectal cancer and CA125 is more useful in ovarian cancer. CA 27.29 is widely used in breast cancer, but has low specificity, meaning that it can be indicative of many other kinds of cancers and benign conditions. Consequently, findings must be confirmed with other tests. CA 15-3, like CA 27.29 (to which it is very similar), can be quite helpful in following some women who already have advanced breast cancer.

However, since CA 15-3 is rarely elevated in women with early breast cancer, it isn't generally useful for diagnosis or early detection, nor for monitoring response to adjuvant treatment for primary breast cancer.

CA 15-3 is sometimes useful for follow-up testing, with a diagnostic sensitivity for recurrence of about a third to a half[9] but because it does a better job at detecting larger amounts of cancer, it is less likely to show elevations in locoregional recurrence than in distant metastases.[10,11] In other words, CA 15-3 will pick up some recurrences, but not the localized ones in which aggressive early treatment would be most likely to be curative. So tumor markers are less likely to pick up those situations where finding a recurrence sooner might possibly make some difference.

From among the many studies that have been done, a Finnish trial illustrates typical tumor marker results, and demonstrates a few of the problems with relying on this test as a sole indicator of recurrence. In this study, 243 breast cancer patients had a CA 15-3 test done every 6 months after their initial treatment was completed.

> *During the five years of follow-up, 59 (24 percent) relapses were discovered. CA 15-3 was elevated in 21/59 (36 percent) of the relapsed cases at least once. The 59 patients were subjected to 199 tests, of which 25 (13 percent) were positive. Among the 184 patients without recurrence, there were 6 (3 percent) with a positive CA 15-3 level. The test failed to detect locoregional relapse or contralateral breast cancer. It was elevated in approximately half of bone-only metastases and in all of the liver-only metastases. In the pulmonary-only recurrences, the marker value was not elevated.*

> *We conclude that the CA 15-3 tumour marker test is specific, but not sensitive enough to indicate the first relapse earlier than other methods. The positive predictive value especially remained poor in patients with a relatively good prognosis. Our results confirm that the test is not suitable alone for breast cancer follow-up.[12]*

Bone scans, CT and MRI

The most common scans used to detect recurrence are bone-scan, CT (computerized tomography, also called CAT scan) and MRI (magnetic resonance imaging).

A bone scan is a nuclear medicine test, where a radioactive isotope is injected that will show "hot spots" (areas of increased uptake) in parts of the skeleton where there has been inflammation, injury—or bone metastasis. Bilateral findings in joints often indicate osteoarthritis or other benign conditions, while hot spots on the long bones of arms or legs, ribs, spine, skull and pelvis may be suggestive of bone metastases, and invite an x-ray or other test to investigate further.

Like x-rays, CT scans pass radioactive beams through the tissue in order to image parts of the body in cross-section. They are very successful at imaging soft tissue and organs, but much less so with bone, or any structure that doesn't change anatomically when it is diseased.

MRI scans do the same thing, using a strong magnet that energizes water molecules in body tissue. With MRI, there is no ionizing radiation, a potentially important issue over time, since damage to the body from radiation exposure is cumulative. MRI scans are very good at visualizing anatomic structure and soft tissue, and helping to distinguish tumors from normal tissue. Like CT scans, they image only a part of the body at one time.

What the research tells us

Several large randomized clinical trials have looked at how well these tests perform at finding early metastatic recurrences before they have a chance to produce symptoms, and then have followed the patients to see if those who received the tests did any better over time.

Information directly relevant to what today's breast cancer patients experience, where these multiple methods of detection are possible, comes from two large Italian trials that were published in the *Journal of the American Medical Association* in 1994.

In the first study, conducted by lead researcher Marco Rosselli Del Turco and his colleagues in twelve participating centers,

1,243 consecutive breast cancer patients were randomized into two post-treatment groups. One group received clinical exams and annual mammography, while the other group received the clinical exam and mammography, plus a routine chest x-ray and bone scan every six months.

At the end of five years, significantly more recurrences had been found in the intensive follow-up group, but there was no improvement in survival as a result of earlier treatment. The study's authors concluded that, "anticipated diagnosis appears to be the only effect of intensive follow-up." In other words, the only advantage of follow-up testing is detecting recurrence sooner.

A ten-year update of this study that was published in 1999 confirmed the findings. The cumulative mortality rates for the two groups were not statistically different: 34.8 percent for the intensive follow up group, and 31.5 percent for the clinical follow-up group. The study authors wrote, "Before intensive monitoring programs are introduced, studies should evaluate whether newer diagnostic methods or the existence of better treatment modalities warrant intensive monitoring."[13] Figure 6-1 presents the update of this study's findings in table format.

Another large Italian study, known as the GIVIO Investigators study, divided 1,320 stage I, II and III breast cancer patients from 26 hospitals into two post-treatment groups. One group went for regular doctor's visits only, while the other group supplemented these visits with regularly scheduled bone scan, liver sonograms, chest x-rays, and blood tests at predefined intervals. After six years, there were no significant differences either in survival or in health-related quality of life, defined as "overall health and quality-of-life perception, emotional well-being, body image, social functioning, symptoms, and satisfaction with care."[14] Figure 6-2 presents this study's findings in table format.

	Total Number of Patients	Deaths at 10 Year Follow-Up
Study group Consecutive patients surgically treated for unilateral invasive breast carcinoma. No involved lymph nodes (T1,N0,M0)	1243	434
Intensive follow-up group Physical examination (every 3 months in the first 2 years and every 6 months thereafter) and annual mammography as well as biannual chest x-ray and bone scan	622	222
Clinical follow-up group Physical examination and mammography as above, with the same schedule but no other routine diagnostic test.	621	212

Figure 6-1. Del Turco study: Intensive vs clinical follow-up after treatment of primary breast cancer: 10-year update of a randomized trial (JAMA, 1994, 1999)

When early detection doesn't apply

Tellingly, 70 percent of the GIVIO study's participants stated that their preference was to undergo diagnostic tests, even if free of symptoms.

Responding to this survey's results, Dr Clifford Hudis stated that breast cancer patients seem to "have a fundamental and unshakable belief that if they get screened and followed, they may be able to get a better outcome than if they don't. That's a big frustration in many ways."[15]

Dr. Hudis could have been describing my reaction, as I read these studies. While the numbers were persuasive, I found it

	Total Number of Patients	Deaths at 6 years (median 71 months)
Consecutive invasive breast cancer patients Stage I, II and III	1320	254
Intensive Follow-up group Exam every 3 months for 2 years, every 6 months thereafter + Biannual chest x-ray, bone scan, liver sonogram, blood tests	655	132
Clinical Follow-up Group Exam every 3 months for 2 years. Every 6 months thereafter	665	122

Figure 6-2. GIVIO investigators: Impact of follow-up testing on survival and health-related quality of life in breast cancer patients: a multicenter randomized controlled trial (JAMA, 1994)

hard to accept what I was reading. How could it be that I had never heard about these findings, after nearly a decade of breast cancer advocacy? Impossible!

I talked to some of the knowledgeable advocates I knew. I asked them if they had follow-up testing done. Most of them said yes, of course, that they and their doctors were vigilant. They felt good about being closely monitored for recurrence. "Did your oncologist ever suggest to you that having these tests isn't necessary? Or that they might not make a difference?" I asked. For a surprising number, the answer was an emphatic, No!

Charles Loprinzi believes that this "unshakable belief" occurs because "well-meaning health care providers have told the patient that they should undergo frequent testing to detect early recurrences."[16]

Both patients and health care providers assume that the American Cancer Society recommends frequent follow-up testing, but of course what they fail to take into consideration is the nature of the disease. Thus, the assumption appears to be: "If we catch recurrent cancer early, we can cure it," says Dr. Loprinzi. "Although this is true for recurrent localized disease, it does not seem to be true for established metastatic disease."[17]

Certainly, the notion that a medical test would not be as good as its promoters claimed was no news to me, having been lulled into complacency by a negative mammogram that concealed a growing malignancy in the dense tissue of my right breast. Early detection certainly hadn't worked well for me, as a Stage II breast cancer patient. But even with everything I already thought I knew about advanced breast cancer, from working on a book on the subject and talking with hundreds of women with metastatic disease over the years, the notion that early detection of distant metastases might in some way be beneficial was hard to give up completely.

"The key thing is that there is no early detection for metastatic breast cancer," said Dr. Hudis, driving the point home. "It's not early when you find it."[18]

Guidelines and meta-analyses

Still somewhat incredulous, I did some further checking. Dr. Loprinzi was right. The American Cancer Society message about early detection applies only to primary breast cancer. The Society recommends no intensive testing for follow-up, nor are these tests a part of any guidelines for breast cancer care.

I checked out *A Patient's Guide: Follow-Up Care for Breast Cancer,* a 2000 update of the guidelines from the American Society of

Clinical Oncology (ASCO), which emphasizes the importance of continuity of care during the early years of follow-up when most recurrences happen. The research that I'd been reading is indeed mentioned, but only in the most general of terms.

> *If you are in good physical condition and have no symptoms, there are some tests that are not recommended for use at each follow-up exam because they have not been shown to affect survival. Some have been shown to miss the existence of cancer or to indicate cancer when it is not present and some are also costly.*

In the ASCO *Patient's Guide,* patients are cautioned to report all symptoms to their doctors, whom they should see regularly for a detailed history and physical examination, and to perform monthly breast self-exam, as well as annual mammograms and pelvic exams:[19]

> *Recommended follow-up by ASCO consists of a medical history and a physical exam every 3 to 6 months for the first 3 years after your primary therapy. Once or twice yearly for 2 years, then annually thereafter.*
>
> *A good physical exam ought to consist of the following:*
>
> - *A breast exam*
> - *Examination of the chest wall, nodes, skin and scar*
> - *Checking for liver enlargement*
> - *Checking for bone tenderness*
> - *Listening to your heart and lungs*
> - *Checking your abdomen*
> - *Examining the affected arm for lymphedema*

The tests mentioned by the ASCO *Patient's Guide* as not necessary for breast cancer patients with no symptoms are: chest x-ray, bone scan, liver ultrasound, CT scan of the chest, abdomen or pelvis, Tumor Markers CA 15-3, CA 27.29, and CEA, Complete Blood Count (CBC), and blood chemistries—although the guide emphasizes that the latter two tests (CBC and blood chemistries) are routinely performed as a part of annual physical exams.

I also looked at a document called *Follow-up After Treatment for Breast Cancer,* from the *Clinical Practice Guidelines for the Care and Treatment of Breast Cancer: A Canadian Consensus Document,* published by the Canadian Medical Association.[20] While no follow-up testing was recommended here either, the Canadian document emphasized that:

> *Patients should be encouraged to report new,*
> *persistent symptoms promptly, without waiting for*
> *the next scheduled appointment.*

Finally, I was able to find a Cochrane review entitled, *Follow-up Strategies for Women Treated for Early Breast Cancer.*[21]

The Cochrane Collaboration is an international cooperative group of scientists and statisticians who employ high quality meta-analysis, a tool for pooling and analyzing the combined results of many scientific studies so that definitive conclusions may be drawn. Often crucial research questions are asked and answered in a series of small studies, whose results are valid, but inconclusive, because of study size and varying results. Thus, quality meta-analysis is vital to resolve research questions in medicine.

In 2001, a *Cochrane Review* on this subject was published, based on a meta-analysis of four randomized, controlled clinical trials with 3,204 women with Stage I–III breast cancer. They concluded that:

Follow-up programs based on regular physical
examinations and yearly mammography alone
appear to be as effective as more intensive
approaches based on regular performance of
laboratory and instrumental tests in terms
of timeliness of recurrence detection, overall
survival and quality of life.

Dissenting voices

Not every doctor agrees with these findings, of course.

Perhaps it's not too cynical to suggest that some physicians may be influenced by concern over the medical malpractice suits sometimes brought against oncologists by patients who may be able to persuade judges and juries that earlier detection of recurrence would have made a difference for them.

Fear of litigation aside, there are few, if any, areas in oncology where the consensus is complete, whatever the research evidence may show. The intuitive pull to test, especially during the early years after treatment, certainly affects doctors as well as patients. Some oncologists feel more comfortable following their patients closely, including testing in the absence of symptoms, even when the research demonstrates this isn't necessary. This may be especially true for patients at high risk of recurrence.

Medical oncologist Bill Buchholz offers this rationale:

> *Patients with high-risk disease might merit closer*
> *follow-up than those with less risk. The intensity of*
> *the follow-up, however, would best be served by*
> *more frequent visits and physical examinations*
> *rather than surveillance testing. Symptoms would*
> *be pursued more aggressively to find the cause. The*

purpose would be to discover disease before
symptoms became oppressive.[22]

There may be some newer evidence applying to a very small percentage of women that supports a broader strategy of surveillance testing, however. In a 2001 editorial in the *Journal of Clinical Oncology*, Dr. Gabriel Hortobagyi, a prominent researcher at M.D. Anderson Cancer Center in Texas, acknowledged that while most women with distant metastatic breast cancer have their disease progress following initial treatment, a few do not, in the order of 2–3 percent. Citing data from an M.D. Anderson database of metastatic patients treated years ago, he wrote:

Some patients who achieve a complete remission
after chemotherapy remain in this state for
prolonged periods of time, with some even beyond
twenty years.[23]

Further small studies have suggested there may be a small group of women with minimal distant metastatic disease who go into a long-term remission (or even achieve a "personal cure") when their tumors are removed surgically or treated with radiation, and aggressive chemotherapy is used.

Other researchers, like Dr. Clifford Hudis, suggest that the positive outcome in Hortobagyi's study could merely reflect the biology of such a tumor, as well as its unusual sensitivity to chemotherapy and radiation. The presence of a solitary metastasis is itself an indicator of indolent, or slow-growing, disease, which could be expected to have a much better outcome. These patients will probably do well, whenever they are treated.

Dr. Hortobagyi writes that if his findings turn out to be confirmed in prospective, randomized clinical trials, "intensive postoperative monitoring to diagnose metastatic breast cancer early should be revisited." However, unless it can be demonstrated that a larger percentage of patients will be affected, this is unlikely to happen.

There is no doubt that the issue of follow-up testing, like so many other aspects of breast cancer medicine, will be affected by future research in detection and treatment, research that continues to clarify and influence our choices.

PET scans

A PET (positron emission tomography) scan is a nuclear medicine test, like a bone scan. You may also see this test referred to FDG-PET, with FDG being the abbreviated name of the radiopharmaceutical injected. A PET scan measures the uptake of a radioactive form of sugar—a glucose analogue—in body tissue. Since cancer has a higher metabolic rate than most body tissue, it lights up on a PET scan, assuming the tumors are large enough. While x-rays, CT and MRI scans reveal anatomical detail, PET looks at a metabolic process. There is less exposure to radiation with a PET scan than with a CT scan, most of it to the bladder as in a bone scan. And, like a bone scan, the entire body can be imaged at one time.

PET scans do not have sufficient sensitivity as a screening tool for primary breast cancer, however, nor are they able to reliably find axillary lymph node involvement, at least when the primary tumor is less than two centimeters in size. Micrometastases are likely to be missed altogether.[24]

As of this writing, PET scans are not yet widely available, are still quite costly, and are not covered by Medicare for the purpose of following up asymptomatic primary breast cancer.

While the cost is high, the research suggests that there are some striking potential benefits for the use of PET scans in metastatic breast cancer. Much of the current treatment of advanced disease has been trial and error, and this shows no sign of changing very soon. This means that patients may be enduring treatments which aren't actually helping them. Changes in tumor size following treatment can often be detected sooner through the use of PET, making it possible to discontinue expensive and toxic treatments that aren't working. This is especially important for women for whom tumor markers don't provide a reliable sign of tumor burden.

Following a technology assessment in 2002, Medicare reimbursement is now available for PET scanning as a tool to follow advanced breast cancer. Overall, however, HCFA stated that the data "...are insufficient to recommend the diagnostic performance of PET in detecting recurrence or metastasis."[25] Since then, evidence from small trials has suggested that PET may do a good job of identifying first recurrence in primary breast cancer patients with elevated tumor markers.

PET does seem in general to do a good job at discriminating cancer from other benign abnormalities, with a potential for avoiding biopsies.[26] For example, it can be useful in differentiating scar tissue from tumor tissue. PET scans can often find lesions that are somewhat smaller than those found by CT, MRI or x-ray studies. PET scans help decide where to biopsy, and to help evaluate what should be done when other tests, such as tumor markers, show abnormalities. Studies have suggested that while the sensitivity of PET is similar to that of conventional bone scans in finding bone metastases overall, bone scans are still superior at finding smaller bone metastases and are cheaper and faster.

Of course, PET scans can also be used to reassure anxious patients.

Because of the aggressive tumor pathology in her case, Marjorie and her oncologist had agreed on her having a follow-up CT scan a year after her treatment had ended. Because there were some unusual findings in her lung, it was suggested to her that she wait for two months, then have another CT scan to see if anything changed. She found the prospect of waiting intolerable.

> I went for the one-year scans and "suspicious" areas in my lungs were noted on the CT scan. Knowing this created an avalanche of anxiety. Waiting eight weeks for a follow up CT scan of my lungs wasn't acceptable. In light of my previous experience, waiting and wondering just doesn't make sense. I'm very aware that it usually doesn't matter when metastases are found in terms of overall survival outcomes but the idea of anything possibly being wrong in my lungs and not knowing if the cancer was there was unbearable. There simply isn't any area of comfort I can find in not knowing.

As it happened, her brother-in-law had just had a PET scan to stage his esophageal cancer, and so she knew about the test and its effectiveness. A short while after persuading her insurance carrier to cover the PET, she had her results: all clear.

> The relief I felt from these results was incredible…For the first time since I've heard the words, "It's malignant," I'm feeling a sense of peace about my current health status as truly N.E.D.

Of course, the need for Marjorie's PET scan followed from her ambiguous CT findings, just as the need for my liver MRI had been created by incidental findings in the ultra-fast CT scan of the heart that I'd had. Tests do beget tests. Neither of us had symptoms, but once the first test was performed, and yielded some findings of concern, the second became unavoidable.

Chances are, PET scans will be marketed to anxious post-treatment breast cancer patients as a means for offering reassurance of disease-free status, and to find metastatic disease early, prior to any symptoms developing.

However, there is no evidence that finding first recurrence earlier with routine PET scans—or with a combination of other tests, like tumor markers and PET scans—would bring about any improvement in survival or quality of life for breast cancer patients. So far, at least, it seems unlikely that this new technology has any potential to change these findings.

Indeed, the results of a successful PET-led search for metastases will be the same as the results of the testing described earlier in this chapter. In both cases, the ultimate diagnostic result is metastatic breast cancer. There is no difference in that situation if a PET scan, as opposed to older scanning technologies, finds it.

Scientific evidence aside, some doctors will undoubtedly choose to follow their patients with PET scans, and some patients will request these tests on a routine basis. But whether this practice becomes widespread depends in large part on the availability of the technology, how aggressively it is promoted, and the willingness of insurers to pay.

The costs of vigilance

A 2000 article on the effectiveness of follow-up testing in the *Journal of the National Cancer Institute* cited a study performed by Dr. Arti Hurria, then Chief Medical Oncology Fellow, now an attending physician at the Breast Cancer Medicine Service at Memorial Sloan-Kettering Cancer Center in New York City. Dr. Hurria analyzed the outcomes of follow-up tests used in managing 786 primary breast cancer patients at his hospital. From the 502 X-rays and 160 CT scans that 297 of these patients received, only two metastases were found, one through a chest x-ray and one by CT scan. Only one of these patients had no symptoms.[27] This is a "discovery" rate of about a third of one percent—a dismal showing, even disregarding the question of whether that one patient benefited in any way from having her recurrence found sooner.

While the most obvious message in this study is that these tests just don't work very well, to my mind, by far the most relevant issue here is that nineteen of these patients had findings in their chest x-rays that led to further testing, including CT and bone scans and EKGs, and all nineteen turned out to be false positives.[28]

I feel for these nineteen women in Dr. Hurria's study. Of course they must have been immensely relieved by the ultimately negative findings, but my own experience gives me some idea of the emotional toll this testing cycle must have taken on these patients. Maybe you've been there, too.

Not included in the research reports about the effectiveness of follow-up testing are discussions on the emotional costs of testing: the anguish of waiting for test results, and the impact of knowing sooner that one has an incurable disease. However urgent the need for reassurance may be, maintaining vigilance after completing treatment has real drawbacks that we almost never hear about. White-knuckling it through the months and years after treatment ends is only reinforced by the belief that testing will somehow "catch it early enough" to make a difference in survival. If there is no evidence to support this belief— and it appears there is none—then the emotional costs hardly seem worth it, let alone the expense and invasive nature of some of the testing.

Yet Dianne's response, below, was typical of what so many women believe about testing and vigilance. She had so far refused these tests, but equated her reaction with cowardice.

> *I've had several people ask me if I would want*
> *a PET scan or a Vitascan. My reaction is always,*
> *"Only if it came back okay!" If I could know ahead*
> *of time it would show me to be cancer free, I'd do it*
> *in a heartbeat (so I could stop worrying) but I'm*
> *too much of a chicken to do it otherwise. This drives*
> *me nuts, because I see how absurd it is. When I'm*
> *feeling really good, I think, "Okay, I'll set up an*
> *appointment!" Then something will happen that*
> *makes me feel yucky and I'll think "No way,*
> *José!"*

In the light of what we're saying here, it's very possible that through her avoidance, Dianne may actually have spared herself unnecessary suffering.

Dr. Charles Loprinzi of the Mayo Clinic emphasizes this point.

> *It is often claimed that follow-up surveillance*
> *tests can be reassuring for patients, and this may be*
> *true if all the tests are completely normal every*
> *time…is it reassuring for a patient to hear that "the*
> *liver test is a little elevated (a couple points above*
> *the upper normal limit) and this probably does not*
> *mean that you have recurrent breast cancer, but*
> *we'll just recheck it in a couple of months to make*
> *sure it isn't going up and more strongly indicate*
> *that it might be from breast cancer and (two*
> *months later when it is two points higher) we'll*
> *check a CT scan next week…"?*

This is the familiar testing ordeal so many breast cancer survivors find themselves caught up in, sometimes repeatedly. Loprinzi is addressing his fellow oncologists when he says:

> *Do any of us even remotely think that this*
> *scenario, which is not an uncommon one, reassures*
> *a patient during these waiting times?*[29]

So, what you're saying is…?

If you've come this far with me, you may be feeling more than a little discouraged and disillusioned. The first reaction women have to this information is often a sense of fatalism and helplessness.

This research on follow-up testing offers a difficult message to absorb, and that's probably one reason why many doctors don't share it with their patients, and why patients don't talk about it among themselves.

As a prominent researcher, Dr. Clifford Hudis is one oncologist who takes the time to carefully explain to his patients why he does not offer them follow-up testing after primary breast cancer. But it's not easy to deliver this message, he says.

> *Of all the discussions we have with patients, this*
> *one can sometimes be the hardest. It's the coldest*
> *bucket of water we throw on them, because some*
> *patients perceive this to be a hopeless situation.*
> *That's unfortunate, because we are not saying that*
> *treatment is hopeless. We are saying that worrying*
> *about recurrence and perhaps finding it a few*
> *weeks earlier does not improve the situation.*[30]

From my own experience, I've found that the ultimate response to this information can be liberating. The initial reaction many of us have is to feel pretty upset. It's no fun to realize we have even less control over what happens to us than we had thought. I certainly felt this way, at first.

"You mean catching recurrence early by testing won't save my life, or at least give me a fighting chance?" Women ask me this, incredulously, after I've presented the data in this chapter in a slide talk. Sometimes, anger will flare, after a despairing silence.

As often as not, the next comment will be: "So, this means if you have a recurrence, you just die and there's nothing you can do?"

Because so many women have this reaction, I want to emphasize here that this is not what I am saying at all. Let me be very clear about what the research actually shows, and what I believe its implications are for us, as breast cancer patients with no evidence of disease.

- Most metastatic recurrences are found and reported by women themselves, or found by their oncologists during the course of routine physical exams.

- Follow-up testing for asymptomatic primary breast cancer is generally poor in sensitivity and specificity, costly, and likely to result in false-positives and false-negatives, which must be further investigated.

- Further testing can lead to heightened anxieties and make it more difficult for primary breast cancer patients to cope after their treatment is over.

- Finding a first metastatic recurrence with tests prior to any symptoms the patient is aware of does not improve survival, or quality of life.

- Although not doing follow-up tests may mean an initial delay of a few weeks to several months in the detection of a first metastatic recurrence, treatment is still just as effective in controlling the disease, sometimes for many years.

- While not generally curable, metastatic breast cancer is among the most treatable of advanced cancers. It is rarely an immediate death sentence, as many patients fear.

- Treatment for metastatic breast cancer has dramatically improved in recent years, and women dealing with it can often preserve good quality of life and normal activities, until very late in the progression of the disease.

- Patients who are known to have metastatic breast cancer should be carefully followed with individualized tests and scans to determine if their current treatment is working to keep the disease under control. This focused testing can spare metastatic patients the potential toxicities of treatments that don't work, and make sure they get the treatments that are best for them.

To summarize, it is not that treatment for breast cancer that has metastasized to distant sites is not helpful. It's only that it isn't curative with today's treatment. Of course, the discovery of a dramatically effective targeted therapy could change everything. But the hard reality is that distant metastatic breast cancer, as we know it today, is simply not like primary breast cancer, where if you catch the disease at the earliest moment, you can potentially cure it while the cancer is still confined to the breast. Metastatic breast cancer, by definition, has escaped the breast and is elsewhere in the body, usually in many sites. It is a systemic disease.

Treatment for metastatic breast cancer definitely does prolong life, sometimes for a number of years. But the research shows that it doesn't matter if the treatment begins before the metastatic disease is clinically evident (has symptoms).

This means that women who have had primary breast cancer don't need to have frequent tests and scans to detect recurrence unless they do have symptoms. If they have symptoms, these should be evaluated right away, of course. This is the most common way (about 85 percent) that metastatic breast cancer is found.

Women who already know they have metastatic breast cancer, on the other hand, should be carefully followed with tests and scans because the response to the treatment they are on needs to be continually assessed.

When I tried to explain all of this to the Breast-Cancer Mailing List, Debbie shared her own frustration with how this information is so often misunderstood.

> *But why don't people hear that message? What I'm seeing, over and over, is that no matter how clearly this is stated, people are not hearing that timing of detection of advanced disease (before symptoms) doesn't improve survival or quality of life. They seem to somehow think it's saying that nothing improves survival or QOL, once advanced disease is found. Which of course is untrue—but how can that message be stated more clearly?*

I wrote back to Debbie that I thought the problem didn't lie in the lack of clarity of this message, but the general avoidance of any real information related to metastatic breast cancer. It's such a threatening and emotionally charged topic for most of us that we have difficulty absorbing information about it—and in thinking clearly and logically when information does come our way.

Most patients in the post-treatment period haven't had a chance to deal with this anxiety in any open way, to think and talk about it and thereby begin to detoxify its emotional effects. They've been given only the comforting illusions of early detection to rely upon as a source of control—or at least no one has wanted to burst this bubble for them. It's easy to understand why. With such an intensely emotional, fear-laden topic, patients want to believe that vigilance via frequent testing is crucial to survival. It is something that women living in fear of recurrence can actually do. No wonder they resist having this belief taken away from them.

Debbie also thought the emotional hurdle of uncertainty lay at the core of this confusion.

> *Perhaps what we're having trouble with is one of the hard facts that underly this issue: There is no way to ascertain whether we are free of cancer. Even the most-sophisticated negative scan cannot give us any guarantees. It's not what we want to hear, but it's the reality.*

Your body will tell you

If you're feeling distressed at this research and its implications, try to stay with me for a little while longer. The process doesn't have to end here, with you feeling out of control.

I didn't set out to write this book with the purpose of disillusioning and terrifying women about the true nature of metastatic breast cancer. I wrote it because I became convinced, through my own experience and that of many women I knew, that somewhere on the other side of the fear brought on by knowing the truth, there is also a kind of liberation.

When I realized the implications of this research, I found that for the first time, I was finally able to let go of the vigilance that had been my legacy since diagnosis. This wasn't easy for me. Being blindsided after a negative mammogram had made me especially eager for extensive testing, as I've mentioned earlier.

But here, implied by this research, I discovered a different message altogether, one that offered a new kind of reassurance—

that this time, I could trust my body to let me know if there was a symptom that should be checked out.

I understood that it was safe to wait for my body to tell me if something was wrong. However anxious I was about recurrence, there was simply no "seek and destroy" mission that would better my chances. I could let go.

Deborah felt the same way, when she read the studies.

> *Given this research statistic, I feel immense relief.*
> *I am glad that I don't have to worry about going*
> *through these tests. I know myself and would worry*
> *myself sick about the scans and blood tests for days,*
> *possibly weeks before each one, to say nothing of*
> *the potent worry time between when the test was*
> *done and when the results come in.*

Nancy S felt this way too.

> *At first, I "counted the days" between visits and*
> *wished I could go in more often than every three*
> *months. Now, I am more realistic and know that*
> *follow-up lab work is usually not positive until*
> *disease has spread quite a bit. Basically, I don't*
> *depend upon my follow-up visits to find anything*
> *I don't already know about or have symptoms of.*
> *When I have had "scares," it has always been over*
> *things I have found myself. I don't have follow-up*
> *tests except lab work.*

Maria W also felt liberated by this information.

> *My oncologist's view is that when symptoms show*
> *up, then we'll look for the reason. I agree with that*
> *approach and also concur that they are a source of*
> *a lot of unnecessary anxiety. Outcome doesn't*
> *change because of more intensive workups.*

Maria B found herself glad to give up the testing, despite her relatively high risk of recurrence.

> *I have not asked the oncologist why he does not order more scans because I'm not interested in spending my time having them. I don't think they increase survival time. Time enough to have them should I develop symptoms of mets.*

Many women find strength in this new understanding, a strength that comes with time, with experience—and with the truth.

For an anxious information-seeker like myself, the knowledge that it's safe to let the vigilance go has been a revelation.

I think it might be for you, too, if you let it.

CHAPTER 7

The People in Your Life

EVERY BREAST CANCER PATIENT is at the center of her own network of family and friends. Both during and after her treatment, she looks to them for support and help. Inevitably, dealing with breast cancer disturbs, changes and often enriches these relationships. New people enter your life, while others may become more distant. Relations with husbands or partners may become deeper and more satisfying, or they may become more troubled, and even fracture under stress. Through face-to-face contacts, organizations and groups—as well as online mailing lists, bulletin boards and chat rooms—connections with other women who have had breast cancer continue to flourish, often for years after a breast cancer diagnosis.

This chapter addresses the profound effect that these relationships have on how women with breast cancer face the future and their fears of metastatic breast cancer. How do the people in your life respond to the risk of recurrence, and your sense that your life has changed? Do you discuss your fears with them, or try not to worry them? Have you found comfort and support in talking with other survivors? What is it like for you when a woman you know has a recurrence, or dies from breast cancer?

Pillow talk

A diagnosis of breast cancer puts enormous strain on any marriage or committed relationship. In addition to the concern husbands and partners feel for the women they love, and the inevitable anxieties about the future that accompany a cancer diagnosis, they often must shoulder additional responsibilities at home, with children and other family members, while still maintaining a demanding work schedule. Their needs, as care-givers, are often overlooked, an omission compounded by the stoic, uncomplaining temperaments of many "manly" men. As a primary source of support, they often feel the need to be emotionally strong, and are less likely to share their own fears and feelings of loss. Yet of course they are also profoundly affected by the changes breast cancer has brought into their lives. Is it any wonder they long for it to be "over" and for the normalcy of daily life again?

When I asked the women I interviewed how they felt about sharing their fears of recurrence with their husbands and partners, some common themes emerged: protection, avoidance, silence and changes in plans and priorities.

Despite her husband's reluctance to talk, Debbie felt compelled to explore her own feelings on a deeper level.

> My husband and I have touched on it, a few times, but each of us is trying to protect the other, and we don't get far. There seems not much to say—we both fear recurrence, we both hope for the best. I sense that no one who has not experienced cancer wants to hear, nor can appreciate, the deeper thoughts and feelings that arise. Even many who have had cancer do not seem interested in exploring deeply. Not deeply enough to be of benefit to me, anyway. I seem to need to keep digging and digging.

Although they may not discuss her fears of recurrence or mortality in any direct way, the character of her marriage has been changed by the experience they've shared, Debbie reports.

> We talk less about the distant future, about
> growing old together and plans associated with that
> (superstitious tempting-fate fears?). We take more
> time for together activities, right now.

A number of the women I interviewed felt that their husbands had let them know, directly or indirectly, that discussions about their fears of recurrence were unwelcome—until and unless there was a specific need. This may reflect already well-established—and accepted—differences in temperament and emotional communication in a relationship, and may not pose a problem, if the woman has other sources of emotional support that accept her concerns and let her speak about them. Of course, avoidance may also derive from an attempt at protecting the partner—or oneself—from an issue that is clearly very upsetting. For some, however, this failure to share fears may point to a loss of intimacy.

Maria W decided not to bring up the issue of recurrence at home.

> My husband thinks I worry too much about
> everything. He would prefer not to deal with it
> unless we have to.

Ivis reported a similar experience.

> I try to explain to my husband that anything can
> happen and that we need to talk and prepare but he
> really has a hard time with it.

For Vernal, the role of the strong woman, caring for others, remained important to her, and to her family.

> *My husband has this faith that nothing will*
> *happen to me again, so I don't share my concerns*
> *with him or my sons, because they consider me as*
> *being a very strong person and that I can handle*
> *anything. This perception came when I consoled*
> *them after my initial diagnosis with breast cancer.*

Learning more about cancer was clearly not what Deborah's husband was interested in, despite her involvement.

> *By sharing my fears with him. I think it increases*
> *his fear. He truly does not like medical things.*
> *Oddly enough, he is an intellectual, a thinker, an*
> *idea kind of guy with great ideals for the world. But*
> *talk about cancer and his intellectual curiosity just*
> *isn't functioning.*

Dianne reported that she, as well as her husband, had difficulty in communicating about her concerns.

> *I seldom express my fears or anxieties in real*
> *terms. I'm much more apt to throw out some sort of*
> *inane comment like, "My back has been bothering*
> *me for a week, I wonder what it could be?" hoping*
> *that my husband will give me a reassuring answer*
> *like, "You probably just overdid it." When he*
> *responds with, "Maybe you should see a doctor," I'm*
> *always quick to say, "No way!"*

Breast cancer brought the stresses in her marriage to a head at one point, Dianne recalled.

> *We nearly split up a few years ago because he*
> *was trying to ignore what had happened, and I*
> *couldn't. One New Year's Eve he wanted me to go*
> *out for drinks (after I had worked for more than 10*

> *hours on an intense deadline at work) I said I was*
> *too tired. His response was "You're no fun, now that*
> *you've had breast cancer!" Well, he knew the*
> *minute it came out that this was* huge. *Long story*
> *short, I even filed for divorce, but eventually we*
> *were able to talk our way through the issue (and*
> *others that were causing us problems as well!).*

Ellen found there were limits to how much she could share with her partner.

> *I certainly discuss my fears with my partner.*
> *She can only tolerate a certain amount at a time.*
> *She then becomes anxious for us/me. We've been*
> *looking for a support group for lesbian couples:*
> *most of the support groups for partners/spouses are*
> *composed of men.*

Worries aside, husbands and partners may simply become tired of hearing about the disease, as Marjorie pointed out. Her involvement with a support organization has made breast cancer central in her life.

> *My poor husband can't escape the topic of breast*
> *cancer. I make an effort to avoid the topic in social*
> *situations unless someone else brings it up. We've*
> *become the poster couple of coping with breast*
> *cancer among those we know.*

Marjorie's instinct has been to protect her husband from the worries that preoccupy her.

> *I've never kept secrets from my husband, but I've*
> *recently decided not to drag him into the pits of fear*
> *with me until I know for certain that there's*
> *something seriously abnormal going on.*

Kate also tried to protect her husband when she could, over his strong objections.

> When I am faced with symptoms that must be
> explored—lumps, discharge, cough—then I talk
> about the possibilities of recurrence with my
> husband. However, he has been through so much
> with my cancers. Breast cancer is only one of them.
> I have lived with cancer for twenty years, and he
> has been part of that long and bumpy experience.
> So, I try not to worry him unnecessarily, although
> he was very angry when I didn't tell him about the
> lump I found five years ago. He doesn't want to be
> protected. He says that we are in this together.

Some marriages appear to deepen and become more intimate with the sharing of concerns about serious illness. A new degree of tenderness and connectedness can develop, in the face of these fears. Bonnie became involved with providing support to other patients, but was always able to share her concerns with her husband.

> What's interesting is that my husband has
> become a source of information and comfort for
> many people. One of his colleagues talked to him
> frequently in the months before his wife's death
> from metastatic breast cancer, and other colleagues
> who know my history have talked to him about
> their own experiences with cancer.

For Nancy O, sharing and exploring her concerns with her husband became an important part of dealing with them.

> Trying to keep my fears a secret makes them too
> powerful. Expressing them helps me to reason my
> way through them…or at least put them on notice.

Sharon B's husband is a physician, though not in the field of breast cancer. She was always able to discuss her worries with him.

> He is the one person who has been through it all with me. He is empathetic and mature. I find that if I share my fears with my girlfriends or sisters, the conversation that follows is more about their fears than about mine.

Families and friends

Women who have breast cancer are often surprised and disturbed by the reactions of the people in their lives. While some family members and friends willingly and quite unexpectedly step up to the plate and offer their help and support, others can say inappropriate and even hurtful things, or withdraw for long periods of time. At such a vulnerable point in life, feelings can be deeply hurt by this. Of course, the charitable explanation is that withdrawal occurs when people are unable to manage their own fears which have been activated by the cancer in a friend or family member. But slights like this are not easily forgiven or forgotten.

Every cancer patient is likely to receive unsolicited advice about alternative treatments from someone they know who is just trying to be helpful. Most of us have to field inane or insensitive comments from acquaintances who can't think of what else to say. By the time we're done with our treatment, we are usually deeply tired of the meaningful sympathetic looks of those acquaintances who take our hands and ask, "How are you?" Sometimes we reassure others, sometimes we try to educate them, and sometimes we find it easier to just say the socially expedient thing.

Not wanting to have to cope with the reactions of others is one important reason women may choose not to talk about their feelings to their families and friends. Emma found that her friends responded in different ways, depending upon their own life experiences.

> Some friends were great about letting me feel what I feel. Others wanted to reassure and gloss over things, change the subject. Everyone who's a "civilian" wants to cover up the issue, move on, gloss it over, put a pretty facade on it, and send it packing. They are uneasy with it, don't understand the emotions, think it should all be over when treatment is over. Which of course it's not! I also believe they don't want to hear it, and do want to back away. They seem to feel that it's important to reassure me. I understand this. But the reality is that I'm dealing with an illness that kills a lot of people, and it might kill me. Putting a cute little smiley face on it doesn't cut it.

Ivis felt unable to discuss her fears freely with her family.

> Ever heard of the ostrich? My family freaks out whenever I mention anything.

Barbara actually found herself cataloguing the differing responses.

> You have the people who are so good at talking about difficult subjects, who, even if you're barely an acquaintance, take the time to listen and respond with kind, supportive words. I wish I were that kind of person myself, because I usually find myself tongue-tied when the roles are reversed.
>
> Then there are the people who just want you to tell them you're fine. They insist on it. And if you

*try to tell them you may not be, they keep insisting.
I don't want to tell them to make them feel sorry for
me; I just hate for people to operate under
misconceptions.*

*Some people are just adamant about insisting
that you are FINE!!! "But didn't they tell you if they
got it all? But you're okay now, aren't you? You're
fine now, right? You don't need any more chemo, do
you?"*

*What they are is blissfully ignorant of what it
means to have breast cancer, exactly the same way
I was before I was diagnosed with my recurrence
(invasive cancer after DCIS). But they don't want
to be informed, either.*

Irene found similar reactions with the people in her life, but
tried not to take them too personally.

*I noticed very early on that my husband, children,
family and close friends can only hear so much before
they become glazed over or just too uncomfortable.*

Of course, it's not only family and friends who avoid the disturbing discussions. Sometimes it's the patient herself who puts an
upbeat face on things at times when she's far from cheerful, in an
effort to shelter others from upset or to preserve her privacy. The
women I interviewed were clearly protective of their children,
and of some other family members, as Marjorie pointed out.

*I shield my family from news until it's important
to share it. I'm the youngest of my siblings and they
worried about me endlessly during treatment.*

For Barbara, this strategy made real sense for her family, who
had been through quite enough trauma already.

> *I think we've all agreed there's no point ruining
> today by worrying about tomorrow. Especially since
> my children are so young, I don't want them living
> through years of gloom and doom and despair and
> fear. They had enough of it for one year to last a
> lifetime.*

For many of the same reasons, Deborah chose carefully what she would share with her four daughters.

> *They are glad the treatments are done, that my
> hair is growing back, that it all wasn't so bad and
> I'm here, not much changed, to prove it. I don't
> think they think about recurrence at all and I don't
> talk about it to them.*

Because Debbie's children were older, they understood more about breast cancer, and she was not as worried about protecting them.

> *My children want badly to believe I'm cured, but
> still express anxiety at times. "If there's anything
> bad happening, I want to know it," my 21-year-old
> daughter says occasionally.*

Vernal's children were also aware that her cancer could recur.

> *My sons ask about my health periodically, and
> when my next checkup is. I know there is a fear
> that I will get this again.*

Bonnie's grown children had been involved with cancer over the years since her diagnosis, but seemed no longer to be fearful for her.

> *I've felt so good for so long, I think they expect
> me to live forever. While our children were very*

> happy to hear that the likelihood of IBC
> (inflammatory breast cancer) recurring diminishes
> significantly after about three years, no one in this
> family is completely relaxed. Our youngest
> daughter works for the American Cancer Society in
> Albany and we've all taken part in Relay for Life
> events, support other cancer-related initiatives, and
> often e-mail information about new therapies or
> other reasons to be optimistic to each other.

And of course, family members who might themselves be at risk are particularly sensitive to any such discussion, and may bring a heavy set of agendas and expectations when they come for a visit, as Sharon B pointed out.

> My sisters are older than I am. They are
> obviously very concerned about their own futures.
> They want me to be "cured" and cheerful.

Deborah had a unique perspective, both as a family member, since one of her sisters was diagnosed six years before she was, and as a breast cancer patient herself.

> I discuss fears with my sister because she's "been
> there, done that." I discuss my fears with some of
> my "non-BC" sisters as well, but I realize that they
> are on the other side and I don't really want to
> burden them. I remember what it was like before
> my diagnosis when Maria would talk about it.
> There was a part of me that just didn't want to hear
> about it. It was a fear thing. I thought she was
> being a bit too involved with it, too wrapped up in
> her breast cancer, and I wanted her to just move on
> and not worry so much, not dwell on it. Now that
> I'm on the other side with her, I understand so
> much more.

While Ellen's family did not have unrealistic perceptions of her illness, she found that being a physician sometimes got in the way. Because they were used to turning to her as a medical authority, that didn't leave much room for her own needs from them, when she herself was ill.

> My family (particularly my sister and brother)
> has experienced serious illness and by and large
> accepts human mortality. Consequently, my current
> situation doesn't seem unusual to them. I would like
> more support from them but they keep putting me
> in the doctor role, which I try to avoid.

Of course, women who live alone, and have families who are distant or uninvolved face special fears and challenges, as Barbie said.

> They consider me cured and want to hear
> nothing from me. Perhaps that is because I am
> single and they are happy that I am cancer free.

For Nancy M, who also copes with mental illness, dread of recurrence was very much tied up with a fear of poverty and isolation.

> Who would be there if I got very sick with
> recurrence? Who would help with practical things
> of daily living, who would be my ear, who would go
> to doctors' appointments with me, and so on? No
> one, of course. Real life is that support from cousins
> and friends cannot be sustained in an intense way
> for very long, and you would not want them to.
> They have their own busy lives. If I was very
> chronically sick, I would likely have to give up my
> life entirely and go to a subsidized nursing or care
> home. You might as well say, I would give up my
> life as there would be no quality for me in it.

Common ground: Finding support in the breast cancer community

The majority of the women I interviewed saw their breast cancer support communities as the primary source of emotional and informational help during the difficult months and years after their treatment ended.

These support communities are diverse in nature, from face-to-face groups, to fellow patients met in doctors' waiting rooms, to sisters or friends who share a diagnosis, to other cancer patients, to on-line groups of all kinds, including bulletin boards and mailing lists, and to many kinds of support organizations and advocacy groups where women and their families gather formally and informally. Anywhere that women who have had breast cancer can meet, share their stories and help one another, seems to satisfy a deep need for connection, especially during the difficult post-treatment period.

Nancy O describes what often happens when women get together.

> We talk a lot about our worries at the Breast
> Resource Center. Sometimes we laugh, sometimes
> we hug each other.

For Debbie, reaching out for support meant going against her own very private nature. One day, browsing the Internet, she happened on the Breast-Cancer Mailing list. She typed an email message, asking for information.

> I've always been a fairly solitary, self-contained
> sort. I've never joined a group, and form close
> friendships slowly. After receiving so many

*wonderful, warm responses to my first list-
question, I sat at the computer and bawled
(and I'm not much of a weeper, usually). Tears
of relief, and catharsis, to find other normal,
vibrant women, thinking and feeling so much like
me. The practical tips and information have been
very helpful. But most important to me has been
the opportunity to explore the thoughts and
growth that have arisen in the process of dealing
with breast cancer. I enjoy the diversity of the
list.*

*I've made "kindred spirit" connections with
many. And as I progressed from the initial "deer-
in-the-headlights" phenomenon of early diagnosis,
to a better understanding of the effects of this
disease, both physically and spiritually, I've gotten
great satisfaction from being able to reply privately
to others in need of help or encouragement.*

Maria B described this mailing list as a "resilient net."

*On the list are people I can trust, with whom
I can be myself—I can rant and rave and worry
and be silly, and lose my temper and practice
forbearance and love these people. I am bonded.
We are like the Three Musketeers—except there
are hundreds of us.*

Emma felt that way about the list, too.

*Being on-line has been a lifesaver. I find it's also
useful to take turns being the helper and the helpee,
so to speak. I've realized I'm not the only person
undergoing these feelings and experiences. It helps
not to feel so alone or isolated.*

Support through the Internet can meet unusual needs. People who are isolated geographically, or by illness, disability or other circumstance can make connections not otherwise possible.

Internet-based support groups can help people with rare forms of the disease connect with one another. For Bill, as a male breast cancer patient, an online group was the only option available. There, he found acceptance, as well as other men with breast cancer he was able to meet and get to know online.

> *The on-line group has been the most help to me. I could not find a support group that welcomed men.*

Bonnie was able to find other women who shared her diagnosis of inflammatory breast cancer, a rare and aggressive form of the disease that afflicts only three percent of diagnosed patients. In addition to the Inflammatory Breast Cancer mailing list, she helped to establish a regional group that meets in person on a regular basis, with members traveling from neighboring states.

Stoic by nature, Francine said that she does not really share her worries with anyone, and would not have sought out a face-to-face support group. But she found support by reading email messages from people she came to know online.

> *While I don't talk, I find it helpful to hear what other women have to say on the Breast-Cancer List. It's nice to know one isn't alone or crazy. Reassuring.*

For Kate, her in-person support group was crucial at first.

> *My weekly face-to-face cancer support group literally saved my life when I was trying to cope with both colon cancer and breast cancer. They gave me a safe place to talk and to cry. They urged me to take control of my treatment, fire a sloppy oncologist, and get medication for depression.*

With all of Kate's health issues, however, attendance became increasingly problematic.

> *When it became too difficult for me to drive into town for meetings, I connected with an Internet support group that provided lots of information and emotional strength. I now manage an e-mail list for colon cancer survivors and spend time each day responding to members' needs.*

An innovative writing program at a local medical center provided not only support but also a creative outlet for Françoise.

> *Our medical center is affiliated with a college of medicine. In recent years medical students from the college have met with our support group annually and conducted writing sessions. The sessions are therapeutic for the survivors and educational for the medical students. The poems are shared and discussed that evening. Some of the poems are then published in the literary journal produced by the humanities department. Then, if the survivors want to, they can read their work to the whole community—medical and local—at the literary journal's annual reception.*

Marjorie found real satisfaction in giving back some of what she has received at her local support organization.

> *I am involved in both on a personal and volunteer basis. Sharing the experience and every facet of it helps others and strengthens me. I think I've been able to help many women by listening and telling them about my highs and lows. Those who were there for me, both on line and in person, were of enormous value in some very desperate times. It goes full circle.*

While many support groups are peer led, Ellen's experience indicates how important a trained facilitator can be for a group.

> I was in a formal post-treatment therapy group at Memorial Sloan-Kettering Cancer Center after my treatment ended there. I was in a leaderless support group for two years after that. It was composed of some of the same women, but I found that much less useful. I would join a support group as I have before but I don't do well in groups that are not professionally led. Since I have an M.D. and am a therapist, everyone puts me in the position of group leader and doesn't let me be a member.

Support groups are not for everyone, as Dianne's experience showed.

> I was in a support group early on but the women kept dying and it was just too close to home for me. I found my "solace" in writing a humor column for a breast cancer website. The writing has allowed me to explore my fears and I get emails from women sharing their stories so it's very therapeutic for me!

Some women, like Vernal, seek out and find other communities of support.

> I did not join a support group with other breast cancer patients, but I did join a Bible study group that I became very close with that I was able to share my concerns and feelings. Some of the women in the group I soon found had either had breast cancer or some other cancers. We were able to share with each other at any time. We even knew

when each other's next appointments would be, and
we would pray for a favorable outcome for check-
ups and tests.

One day, it could be me

Her support group was discussing their fears about the cancer coming back on the day that Françoise wrote this poem.

Talking about Recurrence
eyes dart

necks stiffen

feet tap, tap, tap

who's next?

When women with breast cancer become close with one another over time, they are bound to be exposed to recurrence in people they have come to care about. It's one of the inevitabilities of support groups that stay together, and for many, it's hard not to feel more at risk.

Barbara expressed what is probably the most common reaction.

> *When I hear or read about other women who*
> *had recurrences I get very frightened and depressed*
> *for myself.*

Even if they are not comfortable saying so publicly, many women privately confess to these feelings. A descriptive study I did of usage patterns and attitudes of the Breast-Cancer Mailing List revealed that upset when women had a recurrence or died was seen as one of the important drawbacks of being a List member—and this response came from those who remained on the List, surely a more favorably biased group.[1]

From her work with other survivors and her personal experience, Ivis understood how important it was to keep a level head about this, and avoid comparisons with other patients.

> *I believe that we owe it to ourselves to know that*
> *everyone's cancer can be different. What happens*
> *to one person may not happen to another.*

Beyond the fear and sadness evoked when a "breast friend" has a recurrence, many women find that learning more about the nature of metastatic disease leads to surprising insights. Deborah found that when she was diagnosed with breast cancer, she began to understand what her sister Maria had been telling her since her diagnosis, six years earlier.

> *Even though my sister talked about it and would*
> *even say things like, "women can live with mets for*
> *years," I didn't hear her. All I believed at that time*
> *is that mets equaled death. I had no idea that some*
> *mets can be controlled to a certain extent.*

Since some of the women on the Breast-Cancer Mailing List are dealing with advanced breast cancer, those who have had early stage breast cancer read their messages every day, and often get to know them well. For many of us, this isn't the crushing experience one would think, as Sara M related.

> *More than anything it has helped immeasurably*
> *to read of women living long and well with*
> *metastatic disease. I thought of it as an immediate*
> *death sentence before, but now I know that is not*
> *the case.*

Although we may hope never to face breast cancer again ourselves, some of us have found information about advanced breast cancer to be helpful and instructive. Sharon B's response was not unusual.

> *I know that many women become very frightened*
> *when they hear about other women developing*
> *metastatic disease. Personally, the thing that scares*
> *me more is the feeling of not knowing all the*
> *possibilities. I'm intimately aware with the fact that*
> *Stage I breast cancer sometimes spreads (that's*
> *what happened to my mom). It helps me to feel like*
> *I know my enemy. Well.*

For Debbie, real information from real women with metastatic breast cancer counteracted her tendency to construct fearful fantasies of what might happen if her own cancer recurred.

> *My imagination is vivid and what I see in my*
> *mind is always worse than the reality—so having*
> *a glimpse of others' reality reassures me. It's better,*
> *for the most part, than what I thought.*

Ruthe had just received the biopsy results confirming a local recurrence when I interviewed her.

> *Hearing about other women's experiences with*
> *recurrences, and writing articles and making a*
> *video about these stories has helped me a lot for*
> *several reasons. For one, I felt (wrongly as it turned*
> *out), that if I had control over a narrative about*
> *breast cancer, whether in writing or in directing and*
> *editing a video, I would somehow then have control*
> *over the potential for disease in my own body.*

Not everyone reacts with equanimity, of course. During her treatment, Emma found reading about women coping with metastatic disease overwhelming, and left the List for a while. But she decided to come back after her treatment was over.

> *Hearing about the setbacks, the recurrences and*
> *metastases, and even death filled me with fear. I*

thought I was seeing my future. Well, maybe it is
my future and maybe not. Who's to say? But I
made a decision that it was important for me to
stay on the list. Running from fear doesn't erase
fear.

Many women do end up feeling that despite the anxiety and
loss, they gain more than they risk from these friendships with
women who have advanced breast cancer. Kate offered some
insight about why this might be so.

I have watched quite a few friends deal with
metastatic breast cancer. Although it made me
aware of the truly difficult time it can be, I also was
struck by what they learned and accomplished in
the last part of their lives. They taught me about
courage and about living every day. They also
showed me that you can come to grips with dying,
that what initially seems so horrible can be lived
through.

On the loss of friends

If you do know other women who have been diagnosed with
breast cancer, and stay in touch with them over the years, eventually you may face losing one or more of them. My own first
experiences with losing friends to breast cancer came through
my face-to-face support group. Although it has been many years
now, those memories are still vivid.

Our last meeting at the hospital where our group had met
weekly for nearly a year was a sad day for all of us. Within the
walls of that featureless dayroom, flanked by vending machines,
under harsh fluorescent lighting, we'd shared tears, laughter and
surgical scars, told our stories, offered encouragement—in

short, done all the things that women newly diagnosed with breast cancer do for one another.

But the hospital's Cancer Rehabilitation Service had lost its funding. There would be no more meetings there, no facilitator to keep us on track. The nine of us quickly decided that we'd keep meeting, informally. None of us was ready to let go, not then— and not, as it turned out, for many years to come.

In the flush of that commitment, it didn't occur to me that by staying together our group was inevitably inviting an encounter with what each of us feared the most, if not for ourselves, then for one or more of the women we had come to love.

The first recurrence came several months later, when the two lumps near Miriam's sternum turned out to be internal mammary lymph nodes enlarged by cancer. A few months later, the ache in Pat's pelvis was revealed, on a bone scan, to be the result of a metastasis. As their diseases progressed, Miriam and Pat attended fewer of our meetings. A space grew between them and the rest of us, filled with our fears for them and ourselves, and their reluctance to share the realities of metastatic disease. Too soon, we faced the first memorial service, then the second.

We handled our feelings very differently. Penny and I found ourselves drawn to visit Pat and Miriam, and to talk openly about their deaths and what these women had meant to us. Others in the group could barely speak about them. At our increasingly social potlucks, we rarely discussed our losses. For a brief time, several of us were mobilized to action. We renamed our group Tigerlily, after Miriam's beloved brindle mastiff. We joined the National Breast Cancer Coalition, made t-shirts, marched in Washington.

But our activism could not protect us from the profound effect of losing our friends.

Being in a cancer support group means having to come to terms with an unusual number of deaths, or at least the potential for them. And losing someone to a disease that you too have been diagnosed with makes coping with these deaths particularly complex.

David Spiegel, MD, a psychiatrist at Stanford University in Palo Alto, California, believes that such confrontations with bereavement are not only unavoidable for cancer patients who choose contact with others like themselves, but form a crucial part of coming to terms with life-threatening illness, especially for those with advanced disease.

According to Dr. Spiegel, who has been researching what he calls expressive/supportive group therapy in women with metastatic breast cancer for more than twenty years, these inevitable deaths allow group members to address their own isolation, discover new freedom in choosing how they will live their lives, and find meaning by helping others cope with mortality.

Spiegel's existential perspective, with its emphasis on the transitory nature of life, can be difficult to master, however. For women who have had cancer, such losses are terribly sad. Angela was devastated when she lost her friend Rita, with whom she'd grown unusually close after they met in an online support group.

> *I completely shut down for a while. Didn't want*
> *to hear about good news, nor bad news. If I couldn't*
> *share it with Rita, it didn't matter. I had a pure*
> *driving hate for this disease. I felt like a solid red*
> *block of anguish.*

And it's not only anguish many women face, but guilt about outliving other group members. Many support group participants "feel guilty that they survived and their friend didn't," explains

Susan Hedlund, LCSW, a counselor at Oregon Health and Sciences University in Portland who facilitates two breast cancer support groups. This guilt is mixed with a fear that they will be the next one to go, Hedlund says.

These deaths can be particularly threatening for women with metastatic disease or for those at high risk of recurrence. Rasa Lila described her reactions to such losses.

> I quit going to a person-to-person support group because everyone that I had gotten close to died. It made me feel like I was next in line. It was difficult to avoid thinking, "Well, I've had this disease longer than they did."

Yet some women do find a way to cope with the fear. Even losing someone she cares about didn't make Judy want to leave her group.

> It's hard when someone close to me dies. When special people die—and we all are special, aren't we?—it would be easy to say "I can't handle this any more, I'm leaving," but then I realize how much the person taught me about living well and dying well and I stay.

Detoxifying death

Exposure to a feared and mysterious reality—death—can also be extremely helpful. Women may actually find themselves reassured by what they learn, a process Dr. David Spiegel has referred to as "detoxifying death."

> We're so phobic about death. A lot of patients are more worried about the process of dying than death itself.[2]

Witnessing the process in others helps to make what is frightening familiar, Spiegel believes, and offers other consolations, as well.

> *When you grieve somebody you've lost from the group, you feel in a very personal way how you, too, will be grieved. And, oddly enough, that's reassuring.*

When the women in Spiegel's groups become too ill to attend meetings, they visit one another in the hospital or meet at the dying woman's home. In the online support groups I am involved with now, women often share their last months and weeks with members of the group, either by writing to us themselves, or dictating messages to family members—and when they can no longer do this, often a husband, son or daughter, or close friend from the list will stay in touch with the Breast-Cancer Mailing List, share the sad news, forward the obituary in the local paper or the words spoken in a memorial service. We, in turn, share our memories and repost her most cherished writings.

When this occurs, many are comforted by this process, and heartened to discover that people really live until they die. As Spiegel points out:

> *Even the ultimate threat of non-being can be faced with considerable fortitude, and it encourages patients to see others who can look death right in the eye, manage their dread, and live life well.*

Grieving the losses

Support groups often develop rituals that help members come to terms with their losses. Sad as they are, tributes and outpourings of emotion after a group member has died are also reassuring. It feels good to know that people will grieve for us, too, that we will be valued and remembered by others.

In Hedlund's groups, members attend funerals as a group and light a candle at the meetings that follow a death to symbolize the absence of the deceased member. They also tell stories about the woman who has died and walk, in honor of her, in their local Susan G. Komen Breast Cancer Foundation's *Race for the Cure*.

When I lost my closest online friend three years ago, I was able to do a number of things that eased my grief and aided me in recovering from the loss. I sat at Sue's bedside when she was dying. I said my goodbyes, and tried to be there for her husband and children. I spoke at Sue's funeral, and was welcomed as an "honorary member" of her large family. I described these events to the Breast-Cancer Mailing List and gathered their tributes for her family. I reread our private correspondence, as well as Sue's much-beloved humorous writings. And with the help of other friends, I gathered some of what she'd written into a booklet that was distributed at the memorial service the list holds at our annual list gathering, and posted on the list website for everyone to read.

Though I missed Sue terribly, I never sank into despair. Some do, however. Grief should not be confused with serious depression. Dr. David Spiegel cautions:

> *Normal grief is focused on the loss itself and sadness in relation to the loss. But when someone gets to the point where it is generalized beyond that, where people feel they are hopeless, helpless and worthless, where they start thinking about suicide, and they're not sleeping, not eating, and their daily activities are disrupted—this, I think, is depression.*

Those experiencing these symptoms should seek help from their doctors, and preferably from a psychiatrist skilled in working with cancer patients.

On a beautiful spring day four years ago, I attended, at a cemetery in Brooklyn, the unveiling of the gravestone of my former support group member Penny. Fourteen years ago, our group of nine began a journey together. Now we are only six. I will never forget my lost friends.

Anytime we allow love into our lives, we invite its twin, loss. Cancer advocates and survivors who continue to seek one another out know that there's no way around this. We must let our hearts be broken, again and again. And out of that broken-heartedness find the strength and determination to go on.

CHAPTER 8

Advice From the Real Experts

FOR THIS FINAL CHAPTER, I asked the women I interviewed to share the coping strategies that have worked for them, and for any advice they could offer to other breast cancer patients dealing with the aftermath of breast cancer diagnosis and treatment.

Reading their responses, I found myself identifying with each of them as they shared how they'd come to terms with the many uncertainties that follow treatment. This chapter presents their diverse experiences with coping, adaptation and even transformation, through their own words, as well as some of my own thoughts from today's perspective.

Their hard-won wisdom rings with the authority of lived experience. Throughout, there are the enduring themes of time, hope, perspective and the search for meaning. They show us that a life lived with the possibility of recurrence need not be a life consumed with anxiety about metastatic disease and the long-term consequences of treatment. It's my hope that you will find comfort and insight in the ways these people have reframed their life experience, and that, like me, you'll find in their words a guide for and an echo of your own transformation. They are the real experts.

Try letting go

At first, we mourn for the life we had prior to diagnosis, for our innocent beliefs that only good things will happen in our lives, for our loss of control, our sense of the power to create the lives we wanted. Many of us struggle to reinstate these beliefs, only to come to a new understanding: we can only control so much.

Letting go of these beliefs, and mourning their loss, is part of the emotional work we must do as breast cancer patients. Only then does it become clear that our expectations and cherished illusions are a large part of our suffering. Only then can we get on with accepting things as they are, and move on from there.

Nancy O discussed how she came to terms with this after her treatment.

> *The uncertainty was more difficult at first, when everything seemed like an unknown. I never really expected statistics to give me the answer, only to give me some way to compare the risks and benefits of my choices. However, the closer I looked at what was presumed to be understood, the more uncertainty I found. It became clear that statistics and studies provide guidelines, but no guarantees. So I had to decide which risks I was more willing to take and then accept the uncertainties.*

Many patients come to a place of realizing that no matter how hard they try, the pursuit of certainty and reassurance over the future are elusive goals at best. Like Maria B, they locate the things they can control, and take action, and then they work to let go of what is beyond their control.

> *I've come to the point where I don't want to spend my life's time being overly concerned about*

*things I can do nothing about. I do what I can. I
take my Tamoxifen. I eat organic fruits and veggies.
I have as much fun as I can. I am fortunate that at
this point in my life I can work as I choose. I try to
set down useless burdens. I spend time with people
I love.*

Marjorie came to a similar conclusion.

*There's only so much I can do and the basic issue
is control. My fantasy about having complete
control is gone. The point is, I never had it in the
first place and now I know it. My biggest issue is
moving on and living each day fully despite
knowing that cancer lurks in dark corners and
knows my name. I don't have to sit in those dark
corners even though I know they exist.*

Looking back at the years since my own diagnosis with breast
cancer in 1989, it's clear that my feelings have changed over time.
My own ways of coping have been shaped by beliefs, circumstances, connections with others—and most of all by my
involvements with the larger community of breast cancer
patients and advocates.

It has been a matter of gradually relaxing my vigilance and
allowing life to unfold as it will, beyond my control. This has
meant acknowledging my essential helplessness to alter the
course of events, grieving the loss of my childlike sense of forever, of permanence, and replacing it with a more mature sense
of flux and change. This process has happened slowly, in its own
time, and could not be rushed. The work that I do helping
others has helped me transform that ever-present anxiety about
my own situation into something constructive.

So what began as preoccupation with my own worries over recurrence and the losses associated with my treatment has been transformed by time, temperament and opportunity into a full-time vocation—and eventually, into these words that you are reading.

Get the help you need

Depression, anxiety and post-traumatic stress are underdiagnosed in cancer patients, in part because of misperceptions about what constitutes normal suffering and coping behavior with a cancer diagnosis. Experts in psycho-oncology, as the discipline dealing with psychosocial aspects of coping with cancer is called, know that the post-treatment period is a particularly vulnerable time, for all the reasons we've detailed in this book. The Memorial Sloan-Kettering Cancer Center in New York City devotes an entire department to their Post-Treatment Resources Center, staffed with counselors and offering workshops and support.

If your emotional state is interfering with your sleeping, eating, work, activities and/or relationships, help is available for you. There's no shame or stigma in seeking help, even for women who have been the mainstay for their families. It doesn't mean you are mentally ill or neurotic to seek some counseling or take medication during this difficult time. We all have our limits for the amount of stress we can handle. A skilled counselor or therapist can help. This may be a psychiatrist, psychologist, social worker or trained counselor. The crucial factor is that the person you call upon must have experience in working with cancer patients. Begin by talking with your oncologist about how you feel, and don't allow your concerns to be dismissed. Ask for a referral.

Barbara's therapy helped her let go of the sense of imminent danger she had been feeling.

What helped me most was my therapist, who pointed out a few things. One of the first things she said to me was that we all live in denial of our own eventual deaths, and that this denial would kick back in for me as time passed and I got further out from surgery and chemo. She was right. For a while, I had to repeat little mantras to myself, to quiet the voice in my head that was screaming BREAST CANCER BREAST CANCER all the time. I'd say things like, "But for today I'm fine" or "All we have is 100% of today."

But I find, now, I'm pretty much back to my regular old self. Even though I know, intellectually, I can have a recurrence at any point, I feel like I used to feel—that death is a far-off prospect.

Through the process of therapy, Marjorie was able to find a new sense of equanimity and acceptance.

I visited a therapist shortly after treatment ended because I felt paralyzed with fear and grief. I knew my life wasn't over but I didn't know how to move on and I wasn't sure I should bother to set goals. Remaining cancer free isn't much of a goal if you want to be fully present in life while you're here. My therapist had me write a postcard to him as if it were a year later and I was doing what I really wanted to do. That was such a simple thing to ask but it kicked my butt into gear and got me thinking beyond illness. He also made me aware that everyone dies with a "to do" list.

I may die of cancer someday but my goal is not to live like I have cancer unless it recurs and I just can't ignore it. Breast cancer has already stolen too

much joy and energy from me. I gave it almost a
year of my life and that's all it gets. I'm better now
and the term "No Evidence of Disease" should
reflect every aspect of my life. I was a very religious
person before cancer struck. I'm far more tolerant
and less judgmental now but I still believe there's
more to life than what we know in the physical
realm. Perhaps my belief in the spiritual realm
helps me cope with uncertainty better.

Make your own way

Imagine, for a moment, that the various tools or methods for coping are like cooking ingredients. There is no one right way, no perfect recipe. Certain recipes are popular, and suit many people—but not everyone. Each woman will modify the recipe to suit her particular taste. Some will seek out unusual, exotic ingredients, while others are content with everyday, tried-and-true fare. But in the end, each woman must discover the combination that suits her taste and experience. Sometimes several attempts will be necessary to discover the right mix.

What worked for Sharon B, who was busy caring for her two young children, was a mix of existential confrontation and a heightened sense of the pleasures of ordinary life.

I think that it's important for each woman to
recognize what works for her and go with it. For
me, I've tried to come to grips with the idea that I
have a life-threatening illness. I am out of its grip
at the moment. I don't know if it might catch me
again. Daily terror, daily vigilance means little. I
feel that I will have lost too much if my existence is
one of fear. I try to allow my cancer experience to

shed some grace on my daily life. Mostly, my life
has more to do with the average, everyday stuff of
living than with breast cancer. Thank heavens.

In the process of coping with cancer, many women discover strength and resilience in themselves that they hadn't known was there. This ultimately gives them enormous hope and allays fear, as Bonnie recounted.

During the fifteen months I was in treatment or
recovering from my transplant, I slowly but surely
began to believe in my ability to deal with cancer.
When the fears surface, as they sometimes do, I
remind myself that I had once before found the
strength and courage to get through the terror and
uncertainty of cancer and that I have every reason
to hope that the strategies and strengths that served
me so well from 1993 through 1995 will kick in
again if and when the disease comes back.

Give it time

People recovering from life-threatening illness are told the same thing as bereaved people: give it time. That this is a cliché makes it no less true. What time offers us is the continuous flow of normal daily life, hopefully life without further crises or major losses. The passage of time pulls us onward and provides moment-by-moment evidence that life outside a cancer diagnosis can and does continue. With our diagnosis and treatment we stepped out of the flow of normal life and ordinary time for a while. With the passage of time, we rejoin that flow. Time allows us to go through whatever process of coming to terms is unique to us, and to emerge, as we are ready, into something like normalcy.

When I asked for her thoughts on how the passage of time had altered her perspective, Ann said this:

> As the days, months, and years go by, it gets
> easier, but it never goes away.

For Sharon B, it was the combination of time passing and arming herself with information that was most helpful.

> Time helps. I'm less terrified than I used to be.
> I feel safest if I feel like I know what's going on in
> the world of breast cancer diagnosis and treatment.

Live this moment

The passage of time is interwoven with perceptions of the future. Because the future no longer seems assured or certain (as if it ever was!) after a breast cancer diagnosis, many patients find themselves more aware of the present moment, more inclined to cherish what they have now, or to work for immediate changes, and less willing to defer their dreams and goals to some future point.

Nancy O offered this succinct advice.

> Spend more time living life now, and less
> worrying about the future. Expect to have waves
> of fear. They're normal. Treasure the good stuff.
> Where did we get the expectation that life is
> supposed to be easy?

Ivis made the effort to stay attuned to these realities.

> I try to take it one day at a time. I remind myself
> that we really don't have the control that we think
> and that we can only share our love and
> experiences and be there for our family as long as
> we can.

For Ellen, the study of Buddhism, as well as her work in medical ethics and as a physician directing an intensive care unit, stood her in good stead after her diagnosis with breast cancer.

> *My personal approach to dealing with uncertainty, indeed my philosophy, is to embrace the notion of "not knowing." This translates into not projecting into the future, since it hasn't happened yet. The Buddhists have a good name for this kind of suffering before the fact—"false suffering." It isn't always or even often possible to abolish all thoughts of the future and therefore of fear of what hasn't happened yet, but one can try. I find it useful to engage in activities that enthrall me. For this person that means music, interviewing patients/clients, gardening, cooking and entertaining and whatever seems fun.*

Seek the middle path

With time and experience, long-term survivors usually find ways to seek that delicate balance where legitimate concerns about recurrence are addressed, without obsessive worries sapping energy and optimism. Obviously, this is easier for some than others.

As a long-term survivor of high-risk breast cancer, Sandy described what has worked for her.

> *A healthy vigilance is the best approach, not an obsessive vigilance. What I mean is that you should be aware of changes in your body, but not be constantly looking for changes. I think you will be aware of significant differences without constantly thinking about them. Take care of yourself with*

*regular checkups, but don't worry about markers or
extra scans, etc. These things are okay if there is a
reason—some change, sign or symptom—but are
not necessary in a routine way. Take each day as it
comes and deal with the things that you can do
something about. It doesn't pay to worry about
things that you cannot change.*

Marjorie found that she was able to make the same distinction
about vigilance.

*I'll always be a nut case, but the more I move
away from the initial experience, the better
perspective I have developed. I have begun to
recognize the difference between healthy concern
and not so healthy obsessing over my health and
the future.*

Sara M spoke of the possibility of optimism in the face of uncer-
tain knowledge.

*Uncertainty becomes part of life after a while,
but that's okay. In any case, it (a recurrence) might
never happen, and even if it does, finding it a
couple of months before symptoms appear through
routine scans won't make any difference. In
between, be hopeful that it is gone for good, because
it might just be true.*

Go through the door that's open

In their own ways, many of these women have finally arrived at
a state of acceptance, or at least a full acknowledgement of what
has happened to them, and the uncertainty of what might
happen in the future. They have stopped struggling with what

might have been or should have been, in a more perfect world, and are living simply with what is. They've accepted how they felt, and through that acceptance, found the key to moving on.

After twenty years of struggling with four different cancers, Kate found that she had finally achieved a sense of equanimity.

> *Someone recently told me to "Go through the door that's open." I think that expresses my philosophy about the future. I will be ready to walk through open doors rather than bang on closed ones. This has helped me be open to all kinds of opportunities. Shortly after my diagnosis, I moved to a house near the lake and took a new job. I didn't stop to ask whether I would be alive to pay for the house or retire from the new job. I just followed what seemed to be the right path.*

Going through the open door also means acknowledging the changes cancer has brought, and that they're not always positive, as Bonnie pointed out, when I asked for her advice to women finishing their treatment.

> *I would just tell them to accept those fears, and live as full a life as possible with them. There's every reason to be afraid of recurrence. One of my doctors once gave me the following analogy: the first time you are diagnosed with cancer you begin walking along the rim of a canyon and the goal is to keep you steady on that edge; the second time you get cancer you begin to descend and the goal is to keep you from slipping down to the bottom for as long as possible. My oncologist said it more succinctly: "Once you've had cancer you spend the rest of your life on a rickety bridge."*

But you know, I've been on that rickety bridge for almost nine years now—and while there have been many shaky moments and will likely be many more—it's been a great journey for which I am extraordinarily grateful.

Debbie's perspective is that of a woman much closer in time to her initial diagnosis. But for her, too, the line of least resistance made the most sense.

At first, I tried to talk myself out of the fear. That failed miserably. It was still there, and I felt badly that I couldn't control it. Then I just let it be there—examining it when needed, becoming familiar with the nuances—both the bad and the good of it. This has worked well for me. I say, "Yup, there it is." I look at it. I think through the scenarios. What's the worst that could happen, and how would I handle that?

As I've done this, I've gained confidence that if the worst happens, I can deal with it. I would not say that the fear has lessened, but my response to it has improved. I acknowledge that this is perhaps in part a protective mechanism. If I were able to be less fearful, more optimistic, wouldn't it be a farther (harder) distance from which to fall, if recurrence happened? At some level, I suspect this is what I'm thinking. But on the other hand, awareness of the risk keeps me moment-centered and re-examining priorities, which is a good thing, in my mind.

For Maria B, expressing emotion in words became an important part of the process of acceptance.

> *I wrote in the night—all the fright, the loneliness, the feelings of not being up to coping with this dreaded disease. I wrote and wrote and wrote, and cried, and wrote some more, big splashy words like big splashy tears. Only by voicing my fears and grief and loneliness could I find relief.*

Do what you love

Cancer lends a certain imperative to life, but it also gives us the time to make things happen. When it becomes possible to shift the focus away from what has been lost, and from the difficulties of living with uncertainty, one question clearly emerges. How will you make use of the precious time you have been given?

For Barbie, keeping her mind clearly focused on activities she cared about became the key to her emotional well-being.

> *I guess that in addition to not thinking about it, I try to be helpful to women who may be at risk or by doing things in our community. I am on the Board of the Breast Resource Center and love to talk about what happened to me. I think I help de-mystify the disease for others.*

Vernal also found her involvements and interests decrease her anxieties.

> *My worries have lessened with time, because I am very involved with my community activities, as well as being involved with the breast cancer advocacy community. My schedule and time does not allow me to constantly dwell on my worries about recurrence. I also try to be selfish about doing*

> *some things for myself that are relaxing or things
> that I enjoy doing each day.*

For Françoise, doing what she enjoyed meant pursuing her own creative impulses.

> *I have found the process of creative expression
> very beneficial in helping me clarify and evaluate
> my own concerns about my health. Sometimes I am
> compelled to create a poem or painting about my
> experiences or feelings. Sometimes it takes
> everything I have to write "a sentence of truth" as
> I see it at that moment. Concentrating on just one
> moment in time in one of my poems gives (for me)
> permission to rant and rave, hurl blame, whimper
> like a shivering, wet puppy or marvel at my own
> new-found courage. And then back off and resume
> my normal exterior presence—reserved, cautious,
> and always willing to please.*

What you turn to is less important than how completely you engage yourself in it, as Kate advised.

> *Find something in life that is a real passion. For
> me it is writing. Surround yourself with things that
> you love, get rid of anything that takes life away
> from you. I ask myself, "Does this give me energy
> or leave me drained?" If it leaves me exhausted or
> angry, I move away from it. Get outside and walk
> or dig in a garden.*

Although Francine felt she did not have advice to offer others, her words ring true.

> *My personal approach is the belief that the future
> is inherently uncertain anyway and there's not a
> whole lot one can do about it. I guess that's the*

fatalistic streak. Meantime I try to do what I like to
do at all times.

From today's vantage point, I can see how important my own choices have been in the years since my diagnosis. It is mostly the present and immediate future that I focus upon, making them as rich and full as I can, being sure I am doing what I want and need to do, as much as possible. One of the gifts of having cancer, for me, as for so many others, has been this focus on priorities. Because of this mental discipline, I am a far less anxious person than I was before my diagnosis.

It's an odd paradox that so many of us actually end up happier after confronting a life-threatening illness. Perhaps it's that we become less conflicted, less tormented by the opinions of others or by trivial slights and upsets—in short, less neurotic—after a cancer diagnosis. Those issues simply don't matter much anymore.

I try to do what I love. I've come to believe that the only true antidote to the tragic inevitabilities of the human condition is to live with as few regrets as one can muster, given the necessary compromises and contingencies of life

So this is my motto now: No regrets.

Stay involved

A close corollary for doing what you love is to stay involved with people. Many women with breast cancer accomplish a large part of their emotional healing by reaching out to others who are newly diagnosed or in treatment. They find deep satisfaction in becoming the latest link in the long chain of survivorship that supports so many. It is not necessary to become a full-time advocate to do this. It can involve a simple act of generosity, such as getting on the phone with a work colleague or a friend's mother who is newly diagnosed. Realizing how much you have to offer, and how much you've learned, can be a revelation.

For Maria B, a profound sense of community and mutual support has become central to her being.

> *My personal philosophy is that we are all here to help each other, and that I will find my way of coping with whatever comes as long as I am loved and love others. Ask, and you shall receive.*
>
> *Alone, I am vulnerable and weak. But in my heart and memory are those who have coped with terrible things, and I feel they are with me. And my family and friends...and strangers, too. In my time of need, I will not be ignored. I care for others, and am cared for as well.*

Ann became involved with the board of a large cancer support organization, and today works with a cancer research foundation. For her, this connection with others began with her support group.

> *For me, it always helps to talk. Getting to know myself better and understanding what runs me makes me more comfortable with myself and therefore with others.*

Maria W voiced what many of us have felt.

> *Breast cancer has changed my life for sure. Since I haven't let it go, I decided to get even more involved. It's another way of coping for me, plus, I desperately want the causes to be found and real cures to be found. Because I'm comfortable with science, this is the way I want to go, to learn as much as I can, and then to be able help others understand what they want to know.*

For Kate, involvement with cancer advocacy work has become a daily reality and a vocation.

> *I spend much of my time thinking about cancer, reading research, talking to people with cancer, and encouraging other people to live their lives fully, no matter the prognosis. This helps. It doesn't diminish the thoughts of recurrence, but I have no time to dwell on them. I think I have learned to cope and have confidence that I would cope with a recurrence if one came along.*

These women became involved in one way or another with other cancer patients following their treatment, but of course there are as many other avenues for involvement as there are human needs and interests. The crucial thing is not what or who you are involved with, but that this involvement with others nourishes you, and enlarges your perspective beyond the circumstances of your own life.

Find your "new normal"

Wendy Harpham, a physician with recurrent non-Hodgkin's lymphoma, coined this phrase to indicate "the demands of integrating the physical, emotional, psychological, spiritual, financial and social changes precipitated by the illness into the 'new normal' after cancer." In her view, we don't get back to normal, so much as we work to discover what is normal for us now—we discover a new normal.[1]

Over two years after my diagnosis, it finally dawned on me that I didn't want to go on living this interrupted, suspended existence, waiting for things to get back to normal, for the crises to ease and regular life to resume. I'd been busy looking for my old self, but she was nowhere to be found. How could life resume as it had been when I was so changed, physically and emotionally? When the world was so altered? Without knowing what I was groping toward, I'd actually come a good part of the way through the hard work of grieving and letting go of what I'd lost, and of embracing—or at least accepting—the new realities.

I'd felt resentful of those who'd suggested that I get on with my usual activities when my treatment ended, that it would be good for me to immerse myself in daily life, and let go of this sense of crisis. They were right, of course. But like so many important realizations, this one cannot come from others, but has to be fashioned from the whole cloth of personal experience. I had to be ready. It was a matter of timing, of waiting until the release of all these complicated emotions and attachments no longer seemed a betrayal of self.

In one way or another, all of the women I interviewed were exploring their new normal, staking out the dimensions of the unfamiliar territory breast cancer had created in their lives. Despite her disability and multiple bouts of cancer, Kate found delight and comfort in the details of ordinary life.

> I have had companion dogs who have been accepting and supportive, and who needed care whether or not I was feeling upset or tired. My young dog has given me two additional hours each morning to write because he must be walked at 6 A.M. By the time he's walked and fed, I'm awake and ready to deal with the day.
>
> When he arrives and sticks his big head in my face, I groan and complain, but a few minutes later, I am grateful to be out of bed and moving into the day.

> *Finding this sort of gratitude in little daily encounters is part of the gift of living with a dangerous illness.*

Vernal offered some practical advice about seeking joy in your daily life.

> *Take some selfish time to do something just for you that relaxes you and makes you smile (that could be playing with a grandchild, niece or nephew). I find that being around a young child makes me look at the future with hope, that I have a great life, and it has challenges, but so what! Life can be full of challenges, and it is how we handle those challenges on a day-to-day basis with love in our hearts for those around us.*
>
> *My philosophy is to live each day with honesty and integrity. Don't leave things unsaid to those you love, because no one is promised tomorrow. Try not to put off doing things that you want to do because of cancer, so enjoying the blessings of life and fulfilling your dreams with family and friends.*

Turn inward to find meaning

A brush with mortality calls out to the spirit. Whether through a deeper connection with one's spiritual tradition, an involvement with art, music or poetry, or a new appreciation of the natural world, this deepening process can be profoundly healing. For some, this becomes a time of reawakening of an established religious path, practice, community or relationship with God. It may be a time of turmoil and questioning. For others, having cancer offers the motivation to initiate a search.

Certainly, it was that way for Deborah, who sought out spirituality as a part of her healing.

> *The first and most important approach is to look inward and begin or intensify your spiritual quest. Slow down, meditate, find a spiritual advisor, look within. Find out your meaning. And second, educate yourself and listen to your body. Explore all areas of healing that you feel you need to explore.*
>
> *The rewards in this endeavor have by far exceeded any fears and physical distress my body has been through. It has given me the peace and assurance that if the ultimate happens, and I move out of this earthly realm, that I will be able to do it. To fully realize that, and have no fear, is great power. It will never be easy and it does take work to stay centered, but it is there. I am learning how to fully incorporate that into my own being.*

It took Deborah some time and exploration to find the kinds of spiritual work that were most meaningful for her.

> *Don't second-guess your intuitions. Maybe you will explore something and it doesn't click. Okay, then so be it. But after exploring all areas that you feel you need to explore, you can pick and choose what is right for you. You have then listened to your body, explored, and put into place a healing team that you feel can help you. And remember, that healing is more than just getting rid of the cancer.*
>
> *What we are looking for is more than the physical healing we all want for our bodies. It involves all aspects of ourselves, thus a healing*

> team should be comprised of all those who will be able to help you in all areas of your life.

Many, like Kate, find that having had cancer deepened an already active religious connection.

> I had a strong spiritual life before my cancer diagnoses. Now that spirituality is broader and more accepting. I have learned new techniques of meditation and am less concerned with the details of religion. My father's death several years after my diagnosis helped strengthen my belief in life after death, a comforting thought, although I am still very attached to this life and the many interesting and beautiful things in it.

"I have better things to do..."

A number of the women I interviewed were able to summarize their thoughts with clarity and eloquence. Common to their experience was a hard-won ability to transform uncertainty and adversity into strengths and perceptiveness. Bonnie put it this way.

> When I was diagnosed, my surgeon told me that people die from things other than cancer and that no one knows when he or she will die and what the cause would be. I was certain I would die of cancer. Three years after my diagnosis, I learned the wisdom of his words when I fell asleep at the wheel of my car and hit a tree. I came as close to dying then as I had after my diagnosis.

> I would urge everyone with cancer to hang onto hope. I had 50/50 odds of living five years. I am

looking forward to reaching ten years in the not too distant future. And I believe that we all have reason to hope that we will live many years after a cancer diagnosis. My own experience is proof of that.

Sara W found herself embracing the unknown.

The one thing I do know is that we cannot ever know everything; we are part of a "great mystery." I try to practice so much of the wisdom that I've been taught during this past five years—letting go of worry, being in the moment, "carpe diem," etc. I don't always succeed, but the difference now is that I probably catch myself faster when I get off track and I can start over again without being too hard on myself. Laughter and humor are my constants, and I always try to exude positive energy for me, and for others.

Like so many others, Marjorie surprised herself by managing to find something positive in her experience. After all the emotional turmoil, this was quite a revelation.

Having cancer is not all bad. How odd to say this. I mean, it stinks big-time on one level, but on another level, you do learn some things. You can be more selective in what you choose to do. You may even develop a bit of a devil-may-care attitude and decide you can be sillier at times or take a day to goof off, or make some changes in your life for the better.

Marjorie had struggled with issues of uncertainty and control her whole life before being confronted with what she terms, "the ultimate uncertainty." That confrontation inspired her to write about it at some length, and with great insight.

I don't know if or when it might recur and I have come to the conclusion after much reading and research and agonizing, that it probably is not in my control to determine what happens. At first, I said to my doctors, "I eat dessert every day. Did dessert cause my cancer?" And they laughed. I went on, "I'll give up dessert if I have to!" And they laughed some more and told me to keep eating dessert every day, that dessert didn't cause cancer as far as they knew. I kept probing and looking, but the reality is that there are precious few established risk factors for cancer.

So here I am, unable to guarantee that I can steer this body clear of cancer. What to do? Well, I'm still on the planet, and as of today, I'm ambulatory, I can still see and hear reasonably well, I'm not wracked with pain. I can still work and laugh. I am lucky enough to have my husband and child, and good friends. I can take walks and see movies.

So while I'm hanging out on the planet, I guess it makes sense to enjoy some things instead of to sit cringing every day about whether I'm going to die. The answer is, yes, I'm going to die, but hopefully not today or anytime soon.

Breast cancer is tough. Life can be tough. We need all the help and tools we can get.

My good friendships got better. My marriage got better. I'm closer to my older sister. I know things I didn't know before. I'm happier. Someone told me these kinds of things when I was first diagnosed and I thought she was a tad crazy perhaps, or saintly.

But something about going through a potentially life threatening illness trains you to separate the wheat from the chaff, to prune from your life the dross, the unnecessary, the mediocre. You realize, "This is it. This is my life." It may be short or long, but this is it, and darned if I'm going to sit around feeling sorry for myself or waiting for cancer to knock on my door again. I have better things to do.

Resources

What follows is only a partial listing of the many excellent resources available. The web sites below have links or resource pages that serve as gateways for more extensive listings.

Organizations

BreastCancer.Net
http://www.breastcancer.net

Focus: Breast cancer news and research by email newsletter

Canadian Breast Cancer Network
(800) 685-8820
http://www.cbcn.ca

Focus: Links, education, resources, advocacy

Cancer Care, Inc.
(800) 813-4673
http://www.cancercare.org

Focus: Info on supportive care, teleconferences

Cancer.gov Breast Cancer Home Page
National Cancer Institute
http://cancer.gov/cancer_information/cancer_type/breast/

Focus: Information from NCI on medical options, supportive care

Cancer Information Services

National Cancer Institute
(800) 422-6237

Focus: Answers to any question about cancer

Inflammatory Breast Cancer
http://www.ibcsupport.org

Focus: Information, mailing list and support for IBC patients

Living Beyond Breast Cancer
(888) 753-5222
http://www.lbbc.org

Focus: Information and support, conferences on survivorship issues

The Mautner Project
(202) 332-5536
http://www.mautnerproject.org

Focus: Information for lesbian women with cancer

National Alliance of Breast Cancer Organizations
(888) 806-2226
http://www.nabco.org

Focus: Information and resources, support group listings

National Breast Cancer Coalition
http://www.stopbreastcancer.org

Focus: Legislative and policy change, advocate training, quality care

Sisters Network
(713) 781-0255
http://www.sistersnetworkinc.org

Focus: Breast cancer support for African-American women

Y-Me National Breast Cancer Organization
English (800) 221-2141
Spanish (800) 986-9505
http://www.y-me.org

Focus: 24-hour hotline

Young Survival Coalition
(212) 206-6610
http://www.youngsurvival.org

Focus: Young women living with breast cancer

Online Support Groups

A few of my personal favorites. There are many other web-based discussions and chats and mailing lists online.

Breast-Cancer Mailing List
http://www.bclist.org
Searchable archives: *http://bclist.petebevin.com*

A general mailing list on all aspects of breast cancer

BCMETS

http://bcmets.org

Mailing list and searchable archives for advanced and metastatic breast cancer

BCANS Discussion Forum

http://forum.bcans.net

International bulletin board from Breast Cancer Action of Nova Scotia

Notes

Chapter 1: Two Million Strong

1. American Cancer Society, "Cancer Facts and Figures, 2002," available online at *http://www.cancer.org/downloads/ STT/CancerFacts& Figures2002TM.pdf http://cra.nci.nih.gov/ 3_types_cancer/cancer_survivorship.htm.*

2. Alicia Lukachko, M.P.H.Assistant Director of Public Health, ACSH, NY, from a letter published in *The New York Times,* October 19, 1999, in response to "Breast Cancer Fears."

3. Z.J. Lipowski. "Psychosocial Reaction to Physical Illness," *Canadian Medical Association Journal* (1983); 128:1069–72.

Chapter 3: Cure and Survivor: Two Troubling Words

1. S. Ciatto and R. Bonardi, "Is Breast Cancer Ever Cured?" Follow-up study of 5623 breast cancer patients, *Tumori* (31 Dec 1991); 77(6):465–7.

2. T.G. Karrison, D.J. Ferguson, and P. Meier, "Dormancy of Mammary Carcinoma After Mastectomy," *Journal of the National Cancer Institute,* (6 Jan 1999);91(1):80–5.

3. H. Joensuu and S. Toikkanen,, "Cured of Breast Cancer?" *Journal of Clinical Oncology*, (13 Jan 1995) (1):62–9.

4. H.W. Nab, et al., "Changes in Long Term Prognosis for Breast Cancer in a Dutch Cancer Registry,". *British Medical Journal*, (9 Jul 1994); 309(6947): 83–6.

5. L.A.G. Ries, et el. (eds), "SEER Cancer Statistics Review, 1973–1999," National Cancer Institute. Bethesda, MD, available online at *http://seer.cancer.gov/csr/1973_1999/*, 2002.

Chapter 5: Everything You Want to Know About Recurrence

1. Bill Buchholz, from personal correspondence with the author.

2. A.S. Lichter, et al., "Mastectomy Versus Breast-conserving Therapy in the Treatment of Stage I and II Carcinoma of the Breast: a Randomized Trial at the National Cancer Institute," *Journal of Clinical Oncology*, (1992) 10(6): 976–983.

3. American Society of Clinical Oncology, "Patient Guide: Follow-Up Care for Breast Cancer," available in ASCO Patient Resources online at *http://www.peoplelivingwithcancer. org/*.

4. Susan Love and Karen Lindsey, *Dr. Susan Love's Breast Book. (3rd Edition)*, Perseus Book Group, 2000.

5. Bill Buchholz, *op. cit.*

6. R. Demicheli, et al., "Comparative analysis of breast cancer recurrence risk for patients receiving or not receiving adjuvant cyclophosphamide, methotrexate, fluorouracil (CMF)". Data supporting the occurrence of 'cures'. *Breast Cancer Research and Treatment,* (Feb 1999); 53(3):209–15.

7. Steven Jay Gould, "The Median is Not the Message," online at *http://www.cancerguide.org.*

8. L.A.G. Ries, et al., (editors). "SEER Cancer Statistics Review, 1973–1999," National Cancer Institute. Bethesda, MD, online at *http://seer.cancer.gov/csr/1973_1999/,* 2002.

9. I. Kato, R.K. Severson, and A.G. Schwartz, "Conditional Median Survival of Patients With Advanced Carcinoma: Surveillance, Epidemiology, and End Results Data," *Cancer* (2001); 92: 2211–9.

10. H. Brenner, "Long-term Survival Rates of Cancer Patients Achieved by the End of the 20th Century: A Period Analysis," *The Lancet,* (Oct 2002) 360,9340 12.

11. T.G. Karrison, D.J. Ferguson, and P. Meier, "Dormancy of Mammary Carcinoma After Mastectomy," *Journal of the National Cancer Institute,* (6 Jan 1999); 91(1):80–5.

12. Gina Kolata, "CONFRONTING CANCER; Breast Cancer: Mammography Finds More Tumors. Then the Debate Begins," *The New York Times,* 9 April 2002.

Chapter 6: Follow-up Testing: Fears, Facts and Fallacies

1. C.L. Loprinzi,, "Shouldn't We Be Getting Some Tests? Art of Oncology: When the Tumor is Not the Target," *Journal of Clinical Oncology*, (18 June 2000) (11):2345–2348.

2. Lindsey Tanner (AP) "Full-body CT Scans Often Cause Unnecessary Anxiety in Patients, Study Says," *The Canadian Press*, 3 Dec 2002.

3. C.L. Loprinzi, "It is Now the Age to Define the Appropriate Follow-up of Primary Breast Cancer Patients," *Journal of Clinical Oncology*, (12 May 1994) (5):881–3.

4. N. Nelson, "Do Follow-up Tests Actually Help Detect Recurrent Disease?" *Journal of the National Cancer Institute,* Vol. 92, No. 22,(15 Nov 2000).

5. A. Vestergaard, et al., "The Value of Yearly Chest X-ray in Patients With Stage I Breast Cancer," *European Journal of Cancer Clininical Oncology*, (25 April 1989) 25(4):687–9.

6. S. Ciatto, and A. Herd-Smith, "The Role of Chest X-ray in the Follow-up of Primary Breast Cancer," *Tumori* (30 April 1983);69(2):151–4.

7. "Tumor Markers," a National Cancer Institute Cancer Facts sheet, online at *http://cis.nci.nih.gov/fact/5_18.htm*.

8. F. Safi, et al., "The Value of the Tumor Marker CA 15-3 in Diagnosing and Monitoring Breast Cancer. A Comparative Study With Carcinoembryonic Antigen," *Cancer* (1 Aug 1991); 68(3):574–82.

9. F. Lumachi F, et al., "Long-term Follow-up Study in Breast Cancer Patients Using Serum Tumor Markers CEA and CA 15-3," *Anticancer Research* (Sept–Oct 1999), 19 (5C): 4485–9.

10. P.J. O'Dwyer., et al., "CEA and CA 15-3 in primary and recurrent breast cancer," *World Journal of Surgery* (Sept–Oct 1990); 14(5):562–5.

11. R. Molina, et al., "C-erbB-2, CEA and CA 15.3 serum levels in the early diagnosis of recurrence of breast cancer patients," *Anticancer Research* (July–Aug 1999);19(4A): 2551–5.

12. R. Kokko, K. Holli, and M. Hakama, "CA 15-3 in the follow-up of localised breast cancer. a prospective study," *European Journal of Cancer* (June 2002) 38(9):1189–93.

13. D. Palli, et al., "Intensive vs. Clinical Follow-up After Treatment of Primary Breast Cancer: 10 Year Update of a Randomized Trial," *Journal of the American Medical Association* (1999), 281:1586.

14. "The GIVIO Investigators. Impact of follow-up testing on survival and health-related quality of life in breast cancer patients. A multicenter randomized controlled trial," *Journal of the American Medical Association* (25 May 1994); 271(20):1587–92.

15. N.J. Nelson, *op. cit.*

16. Ibid.

17. Ibid.

18. Ibid.

19. "A Patient's Guide: Follow-Up Care for Breast Cancer," from *Update of Recommended Breast Cancer Surveillance Guidelines,* American Society of Clinical Oncology (ASCO) (2000), online at *http://www.asco.org.*

20. "Follow-up after treatment for breast cancer, from Clinical practice guidelines for the care and treatment of breast cancer: A Canadian consensus document," *Canadian Medical Association Journal* (1998), online at *http://www.cmaj.ca.*

21. M.P. Rojas, et al., "Follow-up strategies for women treated for early breast cancer" (Cochrane Review). In: *The Cochrane Library,* Issue 2, (2002). Oxford: Update Software.

22. Bill Buchholz, *op. cit.*

23. G.N. Hortobagyi, "Can We Cure Limited Metastatic Breast Cancer?" *Journal of Clinical Oncology,* Vol 20, No. 3, 2001: 620–23.

24. A. Taylor, D. M. Shuster, and N. Alazraki, in *Clinician's Guide to Nuclear Medicine,* edited by J. H. McKillop and I. Fogelman, Churchill Livingstone; 1997, p. 29.

25. *National Medicare Coverage Policy Decision Technology Assessment,* online at *http://www.hcfa.gov.*

26. S.N. Yang, et al., "Comparing whole body (18)F-2-deoxy-glucose positron emission tomography and technetium-99m methylene diphosphonate bone scan to detect bone metastases in patients with breast cancer," *Journal of Cancer Research and Clinical Oncology,* (June 2002), 128(6):325–8.

27. N.J. Nelson, *op. cit.*

28. Ibid.

29. C.L. Loprinzi, *op. cit.*

30. Dr. Clifford Hudis, from an interview with the author.

Chapter 7: The People in Your Life

1. M. Mayer and J. Church, "Usage patterns, perceived benefits, disadvantages, and quality of information in an online breast cancer support group." Presented at the San Antonio Breast Cancer Symposium, and published in *Breast Cancer Research and Treatment,* (Dec 2001);70(3).

2. David Spiegel, MD, from an interview with the author.

Chapter 8: Advice From the Real Experts

1. W.S. Harpham (1994), *After Cancer: A Guide to Your New Life.* New York: WW Norton, as referenced in "When the Patient Is Still Tired," *http://www.medinfosource.com/mb/mb991221.html.*

Index

About the Author

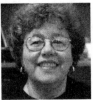 Before completing her MFA in the Writing Division at Columbia University, Musa Mayer worked as a Master's level counselor in the Ohio Community Mental Health system, with a particular focus on groups and women's issues.

She has written two memoirs, one about her own journey with breast cancer, entitled *Examining Myself: One Woman's Story of Breast Cancer Treatment and Recovery*. Musa is author of *Advanced Breast Cancer: A Guide to Living with Metastatic Disease*, the only book of its kind. Despite her own disease-free status fourteen years after diagnosis, she felt it was important to offer a resource for this overlooked patient group, for whom so few resources exist.

After Breast Cancer: Answers to the Questions You're Afraid to Ask was written in response to the many questions Musa has been asked over the years in conferences, workshops and online that clearly reveal women's hunger to openly discuss their fears after completing treatment for primary breast cancer, and gain access to information about risk of recurrence and follow-up testing.

As a nationally known and respected breast cancer advocate, she has consulted for the American Cancer Society, National Breast Cancer Coalition (NBCC), Y-Me, the National Alliance of Breast Cancer Organizations (NABCO), SHARE, and many other national and local groups on survivor issues (providing material for web sites, booklets, videos, and in-person training). She has been a contributing editor for MAMM Magazine (women's cancer) since its inception. As a graduate of Project LEAD, NBCC's science training program for advocates, Musa serves as a Patient Consultant to the FDA Cancer Drug Development Program, and sits as a voting Patient Representative on the Oncologic Drugs Advisory Committee. She speaks widely at conferences and training sessions, and has been active in several online breast cancer communities for a number of years.

Musa also regularly teaches memoir writing, and leads writing workshops and retreats for people with life-threatening illnesses.

Colophon

Patient-Centered Guides are about the experience of illness. They contain personal stories as well as a combination of practical and medical information.

The cover of *After Breast Cancer* was designed by Kristen Throop of Combustion Creative. The warm colors and quilt-like patterns are intended to convey a sense of comfort. The use of repetitive patterning was inspired by tile work seen by the designer on a trip to Turkey. The layout was created on a Macintosh using Quark 4.0. Fonts in the design are: Berkeley, Coronet, GillSans, Minion Ornaments, Throhand, and Univers Ultra Condensed. The design was built with tints of three PMS colors.

Rad Proctor designed the interior layout for the book based on a series design by Nancy Priest and Edie Freedman. The interior fonts are Berkeley and Franklin Gothic. The text was prepared using FrameMaker.

The book was proofread by Marianne Rogoff. Tom Dorsaneo, Marianne Rogoff, and Katherine Stimson conducted quality assurance checks. Katherine Stimson wrote the index. The illustrations that appear in this book were produced by Rob Romano. Interior composition was done by Rad Proctor and Tom Dorsaneo.